O9-AIG-097

Chronic Fatigue & Tiredness

❀ ❀ ❀

Susan M. Lark, M.D.

Cover & Text Design: Brad Greene

Photographs: Ronald May

Illustrations: Shelly Reeves Smith

Printing & Binding: Arcata Graphics Company

Copyright © 1993 by Susan M. Lark, M.D.

Manufactured in the United States of America.
All rights reserved. No portion of this book may be
reproduced in any form, except for brief review,
without written permission of the publisher.
International Standard Book Number: 0-917010-52-3
Library of Congress Catalog Card Number: 92-62128

$\mathcal{W}$estchester Publishing Company
342 State Street, Suite 6
Los Altos, CA 94022
415-941-5784

5 4 3 2 1

To my wonderful husband Jim and

my darling daughter Rebecca

To the health and well-being of all women

❀   ❀   ❀

NOTE: The information in this
book is meant to complement the
advice and guidance of your
physician, not replace it. It is very
important that women with
chronic fatigue have this problem
evaluated by a physician. If you
are under the care of a physician,
you should discuss any major
changes in your regimen with him
or her. Because this is a book and
not a medical consultation, keep
in mind that the information
presented here may not apply in
your particular case. In view of
individual medical requirements,
new research, and government
regulations, it is the responsibility
of the reader to validate health
practices and treatment with a
physician or health service.

Contents

Introduction

A Self-Help Approach to Chronic Fatigue

*A*s a physician practicing women's health care and preventive medicine for almost two decades, I have rarely experienced the health-care problems from which my patients suffer. However, after the birth of my daughter when I was in my late thirties, I went through a period of chronic fatigue that left me wondering if my life would ever function optimally again. Up to that time, I had always been extremely healthy and active. Except for some PMS symptoms and cramps, I had never been sick in my life. Stress no doubt played a major role in causing my fatigue, since I was running a medical clinic and handling a full-time practice of patients, as well as dealing with a new marriage and being a first-time mother. Suddenly, I could barely get out of bed to face the day's work. I found myself overwhelmed with work responsibilities and emotional demands. Regaining my usual level of robust energy and vitality required a major reevaluation of how I was handling my life. No miracle medical cures or "magic pills" could relieve my fatigue or the uncomfortable physical symptoms that accompanied it. I had to pull back from my work for a time and focus on my well-being.

I put together my own self-help program and finally overcame my fatigued state. Today, I have regained and even surpassed my previous level of energy and vitality, and am fully enjoying my marriage, motherhood, and a very busy career.

Learning to Help My Patients

Over the years I have worked with many women who have complained of fatigue and tiredness. Fatigue is a common presenting complaint for many health problems, including stress, depression, anemia, low thyroid condition, chronic fatigue syndrome, allergies, menopause, and PMS. Though fatigue in itself will not kill a person, it can tremendously lower the quality of life and functional ability of women affected by it. An antifatigue program has been a necessary part of the treatment plan for many of my women patients.

Although a woman should have underlying medical problems diagnosed and treated, she cannot underestimate the importance of practicing beneficial lifestyle habits if she wants to regain a high energy level. I have spent years researching the use of diet, nutrition, and many other techniques that benefit health and help prevent disease. I have learned specific acupressure points, yoga stretches, exercise routines, and stress management techniques that provide my patients with a variety of self-care options. My goal with patients who suffer from fatigue has always been to provide information, education, and resources to help them relieve fatigue through becoming healthier women, and then maintain this state through healthy lifestyle practices. Many of my women patients have benefited from a self-care approach to chronic fatigue.

How to Use This Book

I feel strongly that all women interested in self-care should have access to the information about chronic fatigue that I provide for my patients. I wrote this book to share the self-care techniques that I have found to be most useful during my many years of medical practice. I hope you will find this information as useful as my patients have. I also continue to practice the techniques presented in this book. Preventive health care has had tremendous benefits for me; I am healthier and more productive now than I was ten years ago. I am continually expanding my knowledge about self-help and researching new health-care techniques for chronic fatigue.

I have written the chronic fatigue self-help program so that each woman reading this book can select from a wide choice of self-help treatment options. A treatment plan based on only one method that purports to be the only treatment for chronic fatigue will probably work for only a small percentage of women. In my medical practice, I have found that results are much better if I completely individualize each patient's treatment program. By overlapping treatments from various disciplines, most women find combinations that work for them. You will be able to find a combination that works for you, too.

After seeing so many of my patients become healthier, I am a firm believer in the power of self-care. Changing lifestyle habits in a beneficial way gives the body a chance to heal itself. I don't believe that an unfavorable medical diagnosis need be a lifetime sentence of poor health. Unfortunately, finding the information on how to enjoy optimal health and well-being has not been easy for women. Any woman who is faced with the need to handle significant female-related problems finds an almost total lack of available information. Even on topics for which information is available, such as premenstrual syndrome and menopause, most books primarily discuss only symptoms and standard medical treatments; they seldom include in-depth information on what women can do on their own to maintain their health and well-being.

This program is set up so that you can develop your own treatment plan. All the methods you need are contained in this book. They include not only information about diet and nutrition, but also formulas of vitamins, minerals, and herbs, because nutritional supplementation is an important part of an optimal health program for women with chronic fatigue. I have included stress-reduction techniques, physical exercises, acupressure points, deep-breathing exercises, and yoga poses that are specifically helpful for treating symptoms of chronic fatigue. I have also included a chapter on drug therapies so that you can be fully informed about the most effective drug treatments.

Read through the entire book first to familiarize yourself with the material. The workbook section (Chapter 2) can help you evaluate your symptoms, and the Summary Treatment Chart (Chapter 3) lists specific treatments to try for your particular set of problems. These quick and easy tools will save you countless hours spent trying to discover what works for you. Try all the therapies listed for your symptoms; some will probably make you feel better than others. Establish a regimen that works for you and use it every day.

This program is practical and easy to follow. You can use it by itself or in conjunction with a medical program. While working with a physician is necessary to establish a definitive diagnosis of this problem and medical therapy may still be necessary for those women with moderate to severe symptoms, the importance of a good self-help program cannot be underestimated. For many women, this book can help speed up the diagnostic process. My self-help techniques can play a major role in reducing the severity of your symptoms and preventing recurrences of the disease process. Best of all, it works. The feeling of wellness that can be yours with a self-help program will radiate out and touch your whole life. You will have more time and energy to enjoy your work, your family, and other pleasures in life. Most of my patients tell me that their lives have been positively transformed by following these beneficial self-help techniques.

Identifying
the Problem

What Is
Chronic Fatigue?

*C*hronic fatigue is one of the most common complaints physicians hear. In at least 20 percent of all medical visits, patients name fatigue as a significant symptom. Millions of people function below par, accepting chronic fatigue and tiredness as a way of life. They never seek medical care because they think fatigue is a burden that they simply must endure. In my practice, many of the women seeking help are so tired that they have difficulty carrying out their day-to-day functions. My patients often tell me that their lack of energy seriously affects their quality of life. Many women find it hard to get up and get going from the moment the alarm rings in the morning. For these women, doing their daily tasks at work or even interacting with friends and family may be difficult. Many of my patients also complain of losing steam and tiring in the afternoon. Once this fatigue sets in, it may pursue women until they drop into exhausted sleep at bedtime. When seeing a new patient, fatigue is one of the first complaints that I address, because sufficient energy is central to day-to-day functioning.

Fatigue has many causes; it is a component of many of the most common health problems affecting women. When a woman identifies fatigue as a serious complaint, one or more of four body systems may be compromised:

- The *immune system* fights foreign invaders in the body, such as bacteria, viruses, and cancer cells.

- The *endocrine or glandular system* regulates reproductive and metabolic functions, such as menstruation and the efficient burning of food for energy. The endocrine glands communicate with one another by secreting into the bloodstream chemicals called hormones that carry chemical messages from one gland to another.

- The *hematological system* is responsible for forming red blood cells, which carry oxygen to all tissues of the body, and white blood cells, which fight infections and other invaders in the body.

- The *nervous system* comprises the fibers that connect the brain, organs, and muscles by transmitting impulses that allow normal bodily sensation and movement, as well as the experience and expression of moods and feelings.

The remainder of this chapter discusses problems that arise in these systems—problems in which fatigue is a significant symptom.

The Immune System

Chronic Fatigue Syndrome (CFS)

One of the most publicized causes of fatigue today, chronic fatigue syndrome (CFS) has been diagnosed in 3 million Americans. It is thought that millions more are affected by this severe and disabling problem but are undiagnosed.

Women predominate among persons affected with CFS: 70 percent of the cases are female. Fatigue is the most prevalent symptom, occurring in almost all the afflicted. The onset of fatigue is often sudden, and many women can pinpoint when it started. The fatigue is so severe that even minor exertion, such as a short walk or light housework, can be debilitating. The loss of physical stamina and endurance is pronounced in women with

CFS. Many women with CFS curtail their activities and take naps during the day or sleep more hours at night. Interestingly, increased bed rest doesn't improve the energy level of afflicted women. CFS occurs with a whole range of other symptoms, including headaches, low-grade fever, swollen lymph nodes, sore throat, depression, poor ability to concentrate and decreased mental acuity, muscle and joint aches and pains, allergies, digestive complaints, weight loss, and skin rashes.

For many women, mental and emotional symptoms seem to predominate. Short-term memory may be diminished. Women with CFS often have trouble remembering specific names or places, or doing complex mental work, such as bookkeeping, administrative tasks, or teaching. Thus, women with CFS may have great difficulty performing functions that demand intellectual skills.

Medical researchers have found no causative agent for CFS. The most widely accepted hypothesis is that a virus or a group of viruses is involved, although this has not been definitely proven. Most of the attention has focused on the herpes family of viruses as the causative agents. These include the Epstein-Barr virus (EBV), herpes simplex viruses (genital and oral), and cytomegalovirus (CMV). Some researchers have suggested that the causative agents may be *Candida albicans*, a retrovirus that is in the same family as the AIDS virus, or parasites. Some physicians even propose a mixed infectious cause, with several pathogens causing symptoms simultaneously. A wide variety of environmental and lifestyle factors may also contribute to CFS by stressing the immune system. Many of my CFS patients report extreme and prolonged emotional stress, anxiety, and depression, and a history of poor nutritional habits predating the onset of CFS. Environmental pollutants and contaminants may also play a role in weakening the body and allowing CFS to develop.

The length of the illness varies. One-third of CFS patients recover fairly quickly, regaining their health within a few months. Another third of CFS patients take two years to recover, while the other third remain ill after two years. I have seen patients in my practice for whom CFS has been a long-term and extremely debilitating condition. These women had tried many drugs and natural treatment regimens. In treating women with CFS, I have had wonderful success with a variety of supportive techniques, primarily in the self-help or lifestyle area. I describe these techniques fully in the following chapters.

Candida Infections

Although commonly referred to as a yeast, *Candida albicans* is actually a parasitic fungus that only resembles a yeast. Found most commonly in the large intestine and esophagus, candida is a normal inhabitant of the digestive tract and usually lives in balance with friendly bacteria that help the digestive system function optimally. When the balance between the bacteria and the fungi is upset, candida may proliferate, infecting tissues of the digestive tract, vagina, and mouth. The toxins released by the fungi weaken the immune system, allowing candida to penetrate throughout the body and spread to other systems, such as the bladder and respiratory system.

Women with candida infections in the vagina (candida vaginitis) often have a thick vaginal discharge, redness, itching, and burning. Women with digestive symptoms of candida may have heartburn, bloating, gas, abdominal pain, constipation, and diarrhea. Candida infection of the mouth is called thrush and most commonly afflicts infants and children. Thrush presents with white lesions inside the mouth and on the tongue. In the most severe cases, candida can travel through the bloodstream to invade every organ system in the body. This type of blood poisoning is called candida septicemia and is usually seen only in seriously ill patients, such as people with AIDS or terminal cancer.

The weakening of the immune system caused by the overgrowth of candida has been linked to many symptoms other than those of active infection. These include chronic fatigue, lethargy, poor ability to concentrate, depression, visual changes, pain and swelling in joints, nasal congestion, sore throats, and muscle weakness. Candida infections are more common in diabetics and have been linked to the prolonged use of antibiotics, cortisone, or birth control pills. Diets that include large amounts of bread, alcoholic drinks, candy, cookies, fruit juice, and other foods with high sugar or yeast content promote the growth of candida.

Because candida is present in most people, a candida infection is difficult to diagnose. Women with candida vaginitis may be diagnosed by identifying the organisms on a slide. However, for women who may have candida in other organ systems and tissues, the most definitive diagnostic test may be their response to a sugar- and yeast-free diet, as well as their response to the appropriate medication. See the self-help section of this book for more information on effective medical and self-help treatment for candida.

Allergies

Allergies occur when the body's immune system overreacts to harmless substances. Normally, the immune system is on the alert for invaders such as viruses, bacteria, and other organisms that cause disease. The immune system's job is to identify these invaders and destroy them before they cause illness. In allergic people, this system begins to react to other substances—typically pollens, molds, or foods such as milk or wheat (called allergens). Sometimes allergic reactions are easily diagnosed, because the symptoms occur immediately after the encounter with the allergen. Immediate allergic symptoms include wheezing, itching and tearing of the eyes, nasal congestion, and hives. Some allergic reactions are delayed; they may occur hours or days after exposure to the allergen. Delayed symptoms include joint aches and pains, eczema, and fatigue and depression. The person affected may be unaware that an allergy is causing her symptoms. Fatigue is a very common symptom of an allergic reaction; it can accompany an allergy to foods or to chemical or environmental triggers.

Allergies are very common; approximately 24 million Americans (10 percent of the population) suffer from allergies. As much as $1 billion is spent each year in the medical treatment of allergies, while an additional $1 billion is lost in time away from work and allergy-related disability compensation. Several tests are available for diagnosing allergies; they are not always accurate and can be expensive. Physicians don't agree on the usefulness or accuracy of the different types of tests. The most traditional type has been skin testing: A minute amount of allergen is placed on or within the skin, and the physician then observes whether an allergic reaction takes place (commonly a red swelling or itching and tenderness). Any reactions take place within a day or two. Traditional allergists consider blood tests, such as the RAST test (radio allergosorbent test) and the FICA (food immune complex assay), to be more controversial. These tests detect rises in the specific IgE antibodies; a rise reflects the body's immune response to different allergens. My experience with RAST testing finds that it may be inaccurate or not correlate well with actual clinical symptoms. It is also less sensitive than skin testing.

Some holistic physicians test for food allergies by doing sublingual provocative tests. In this test, a food extract is placed under the tongue to see whether it elicits a reaction. Neutralizing antidotes are then administered to the patient to reduce or eliminate symptoms. This test is not used by traditional allergists, who consider it to be ineffective. Another way to test for food sensitivities is simply to eliminate suspected food allergens. First, the patient fasts, taking only distilled water for several days. Then she reintroduces foods one at a time. If the patient is allergic to a specific food, a reaction will occur after she adds that food to her diet.

Treatment for allergy usually includes avoiding the offending substance, if possible, or using over-the-counter and prescription medication and desensitization shots. Managing stress and following a low-stress elimination diet may also be very helpful in treating and preventing allergies. It is also important to rotate foods and choose from a wide variety of high-nutrient food. The dietary principles discussed in this book are very helpful for women with allergies.

Endocrine or Glandular System

Premenstrual Syndrome

Premenstrual syndrome (PMS) is one of the most common problems affecting women during their reproductive years (from the teens to the early fifties). PMS affects between one-third and one-half of all American women between the ages of 20 and 50—in other words, as many as 10 to 14 million women. There is no single cause of PMS; medical researchers now believe that various hormonal and chemical imbalances can trigger PMS symptoms. The symptoms usually begin 10 to 14 days before the onset of the menstrual period and become progressively worse until the onset of menstruation or, for some women, several days after the onset. This means that millions of women spend half of each month of their adult lives feeling sick.

The symptoms of PMS are numerous and involve almost every system in the body. More than 150 symptoms have been documented: emotionally based symptoms such as anxiety, irritability, mood swings, depression, and fatigue, and physical symptoms such as headaches, bloating, breast tenderness, weight gain, sugar craving, and acne. For many women, the emotional symptoms and fatigue are the most severe, adversely affecting their family relationships and their ability to work.

A woman may have as many as 10 or 12 of these symptoms. Many PMS patients describe severe personality changes—much like Dr. Jekyll and Mr. Hyde. They say they are irritable, witchy, and mean—that they yell at their children, pick fights with their spouses, and snap at friends and co-workers. They often spend the rest of the month repairing the emotional damage done to their relationships during this time.

Many factors increase the risk of PMS in susceptible women. It occurs most frequently in women over 30. (The most severe symptoms occur in women in their thirties and forties.) Women are at high risk when they are under significant emotional stress or if they have poor nutritional habits and don't exercise. Women who are unable to tolerate birth control pills seem to be more likely to suffer PMS, as are women who have had a pregnancy complicated by toxemia. Also, the more children a woman has, the more severe her PMS symptoms. PMS rarely goes away spontaneously without treatment. My experience is that it gets worse with age. Some of my most uncomfortable patients are women in their middle to late forties, who are also approaching menopause. These women often feel they have the worst of both life phases as they pass from their active reproductive years into menopause. Often, PMS symptoms coexist with bleeding irregularities and hot flashes. Once the PMS is treated, the accompanying fatigue and mood symptoms clear up. Therapies for PMS are discussed in the self-help section of this book.

No single hormonal or chemical imbalance has been linked to PMS. Instead, nearly two dozen hormonal, chemical, and nutritional imbalances may contribute to causing the symptoms. Even more confusing for patients and physicians alike is that the underlying causes may differ from one woman to another. As a result, no single wonder drug cures PMS, although many drugs have been tested, including hormones, tranquilizers, antidepressants, and diuretics. Luckily, PMS seems to respond very well to healthful lifestyle changes. In my practice, I have found PMS to be a very treatable problem. It does require, however, that women participate actively in their own program, adopt better nutritional habits, and deal with stress more effectively.

Menopause

Menopause, the end of all menstrual bleeding, occurs for most women between the ages of 48 and 52. However, some women cease menstruating as young as their late thirties or early forties, while others continue to menstruate into their mid-fifties. Fatigue often accompanies this process as women go through the hormonal changes that lead to the cessation of menstruation.

For most women, the transition to menopause occurs gradually, triggered by a slowdown in the function of their ovaries. The process begins four to six years before the last menstrual period and continues for several years after. During this period of transition, estrogen production from the ovaries decreases, finally dropping to such low levels that menstruation becomes irregular and finally ceases entirely. For some women this transition to a new, lower level of hormonal equilibrium is easy and uneventful. For many women, however, the transition is difficult and fraught with many uncomfortable symptoms, such as irregular bleeding, hot flashes, mood swings, and fatigue. As many as 80 percent of all women going through menopause experience some of these symptoms.

Many women approaching menopause experience heavy, irregular bleeding. The increased blood loss in these women can trigger a loss of energy as well as decreased stamina and endurance. Though most cases of heavy, irregular bleeding in transitional women are due to fluctuating hormonal levels, other medical problems can cause bleeding, too. These include fibroid tumors (an overgrowth in the muscular tissue of the uterus), polyps, uterine cancer, and cervical cancer.

The hormonal deficiency that develops during this period may also trigger other physical and emotional symptoms. One of the most uncomfortable symptoms is hot flashes—sudden and intense sensations of heat that occur unexpectedly. A woman suddenly notices that she feels warm, and often experiences heavy sweating. As the sweating cools her skin temperature, she begins to shiver. In response to this uncomfortable fluctuation in temperature, many women alternately shed and add clothes. Hot flashes frequently begin on the chest, neck, or face, and radiate to other parts of the body.

Eighty percent of women in menopause experience hot flashes, with 40 percent of these women having symptoms severe enough to seek medical care. Hot flashes may occur during both day and night. When they occur at night, they can interrupt a woman's sleep pattern, leaving her exhausted and fatigued during the day from sleep deprivation. Though most flashes appear to occur without any specific environmental trigger, coffee and alcohol intake may spark a flash. The frequency, intensity, and duration of hot flashes vary greatly. For most women they last two or three minutes, but they can last longer, even up to an hour in some cases. In most women, the symptoms begin to subside within four to six years after the last menstrual period.

The tissues of the vagina and urethra undergo a number of changes as the hormonal levels diminish. The vaginal and urethral linings become thinner, drier, and inelastic. Blood supply to the vaginal and urethral area decreases. The cervix secretes much less mucous than in a woman's fertile years. The vagina actually shrinks, becoming much shorter and narrower at the opening. As a result, sexual intercourse often becomes painful or uncomfortable. Sexual arousal no longer produces the same level of lubrication, and the capacity for vaginal expansion in response to sexual arousal may decrease. Vaginal infections may become more frequent because the tissues are easily traumatized. The changes that occur in the urethral tissues may increase the frequency of urination. Women find that they have to get up at night to void, which—like hot flashes—can interrupt sleep and worsen fatigue. Even more frustrating for some women is the tendency to leak urine when they laugh, sneeze, or cough.

Besides the physical changes, many women may note mild to marked changes in their moods during menopause. These symptoms include insomnia (often associated with hot flashes), irritability, anxiety, depression, and fatigue. Both estrogen and progesterone have been studied for their effects on mood: If estrogen predominates, women tend to feel anxious; if progesterone predominates, women may feel depressed and tired. With a decrease in both hormones, symptoms can run the gamut from irritability to fatigue and depression. The severity of the symptoms probably depends on the woman's individual biochemistry, as well as social factors. Women have worse symptoms if they are under severe emotional stress or have aggravating dietary habits, such as excessive caffeine, sugar, or alcohol intake.

Many effective treatments, such as hormonal replacement therapy and the use of vitamin, herbal, and mineral supplements, help support menopausal women's reproductive and glandular systems. Stress management techniques and regular exercise may also help to restore energy and vitality and stabilize mood. These are discussed in the self-help section of this book.

Hypothyroidism

Hypothyroidism—an underactive thyroid—is far more common in females than in males. In fact, 90 percent of diagnosed cases are women. Low thyroid condition is a common cause of chronic fatigue and tends to worsen with age. The thyroid affects our energy level because it controls our metabolism (the rate at which our cells burn fuel and oxygen). Women with a slow metabolism caused by an underactive thyroid can suffer from a variety of symptoms. Besides fatigue, hypothyroid women often complain of a hoarse voice, constipation, intolerance to cold, thickening and scaling of skin, facial puffiness, delay of deep tendon reflexes, and slowness of speech, thought, and movement. They also tend to gain weight easily and find it hard to lose weight on a conventional diet. They may suffer from low blood pressure as well as low blood sugar and may crave carbohydrates. Clinical diagnosis of hypothyroidism in older women may be difficult because many women do not have the typical symptoms mentioned above. In many older women, debilitation and apathy may be the only signs of low thyroid function. Medical studies suggest that thyroid screening by simple blood tests of thyroid hormones should be a routine part of the physical examination for older patients.

Hypothyroidism is generally treated by thyroid replacement therapy. Older patients may require a much lower maintenance dose of thyroxine than younger women. Self-help aspects of treatment and prevention include taking iodine either in the diet or in supplementary form. According to some evidence, adequate intake of vitamin A, vitamin E, and iodine may be necessary to maintain thyroid health and integrity. Once the underlying thyroid deficiency is treated, many fatigued women notice a rapid improvement in their energy level and vitality.

Women with low thyroid function often have exhaustion in other endocrine glands. The adrenal glands are particularly affected by poor thyroid function, as well as any other physical and emotional stress. The adrenals are two almond-sized glands that secrete several dozen hormones. Cortisol is an important hormone produced by the adrenal glands that helps regulate our response to stress. Stress can be a response to strong emotional feelings, such as anxiety or depression, or to physical triggers, such as an allergic reaction, infectious disease, burns, surgery, or an accident. Whatever the source of stress, cortisol lessens its injurious effects on the body, reducing pain, swelling, and fever.

When stress has been recurrent and of long duration, the adrenal glands can become exhausted, mustering less and less ability to buffer the negative effects of physical and emotional stress. As a result of adrenal exhaustion, the individual may experience an increase in fatigue and tiredness. Much rest, stress management, and nutritional support is required to restore the adrenals and rebuild the physiological "cushion" to deal with stress. Many helpful techniques listed in the self-help section of this book help to restore the glandular system.

Hematological (Blood-Forming) System

Anemia

Anemia is one of the most common health problems affecting women of all ages. As many as 20 percent of all American women suffer from anemia. Women who are anemic have a reduced number of red cells circulating in their blood or a reduced amount of hemoglobin (the oxygen-carrying protein in the red blood cells). Anemia reduces the amount of oxygen available to all the cells of the body, so the cells for the body's normal chemical functioning have less available energy. Important processes, such as muscular activity and cell building and repair, slow down and become less efficient. Greater than 95 percent of the body's chemical reactions depend on optimal oxygen levels in the cells and tissues. As a result, the symptoms of anemia can be very debilitating.

Because the lack of oxygen impairs the body's ability to carry out its numerous chemical reactions, many women with anemia feel extremely tired and fatigued. Because muscular activity is inhibited, they lack endurance and physical stamina. I have had many physically active patients who had to stop pursuing vigorous aerobic exercise programs when they developed anemia, because they lacked the physical energy to continue an active exercise regimen.

When the brain cells lack oxygen, dizziness may result and mental faculties are less sharp. Women who are anemic tend to be pale with poor skin color and tone. They often appear "washed out" and seem listless. They lack the glowing skin color that we tend to associate with good health and vitality. Women with anemia may also suffer from hair loss and brittle, ridged fingernails.

Digestive symptoms include loss of appetite, sore tongue, abdominal pain, heartburn, and diarrhea. In more severe cases, women can suffer from symptoms as varied as headaches, heart palpitations, tingling in the fingers and feet, loss of coordination, and a yellowing of the skin. As you can see, a woman can become quite ill from the physical and mental effects of anemia if her physician does not diagnose her condition properly.

Many cases of anemia are caused by nutritional deficiencies. Without sufficient nutritional factors, the red blood cells cannot grow and mature normally. The most common cause of anemia is iron deficiency. In fact, as many as one-third to one-half of young American women have low or depleted iron stores. The main reason for these low reserves is that women simply don't eat enough iron-rich foods.

Children, adolescents, and women during their reproductive

years are at particular risk of iron deficiency anemia. Children and teenage girls need this iron to support growth and development; grown women need it to replace the iron lost in the monthly menstrual period. This increased need for iron persists until menopause, when the monthly blood loss finally ceases. Elderly women are still susceptible to developing anemia because they tend to eat less and have a nutrient-poor diet, especially if they live alone or have a limited income.

Pregnancy and the postpartum period are also vulnerable times for women because fetuses and breast-feeding infants take iron from the mother. Women athletes also have an increased need for iron during training because of the metabolic demands of heavy exercise.

Some women develop iron deficiency anemia because their bodies are unable to absorb and assimilate iron properly. Iron absorption may be decreased by chronic diarrhea, laxative abuse, or malabsorption diseases such as celiac disease and sprue, as well as by nutritional deficiencies of vitamins and minerals needed for the health of the digestive tract.

Another common reason for the development of iron deficiency anemia is excessive blood loss. This is commonly seen in women who suffer from menorrhagia (heavy or prolonged menstrual bleeding) caused by hormonal imbalances, fibroid tumors, or uterine cancer. Women who use intrauterine devices for contraception are also at higher risk of blood loss, as are women who overuse anti-inflammatory medications such as aspirin or ibuprofen, which can cause blood loss through irritation of the digestive tract.

Besides iron, other nutrients are needed for healthy red blood cell growth and maturation. Deficiencies of vitamin B_{12}, folic acid, and vitamin B_6 are also common causes of anemia. Vitamin E is important for red blood cell survival. Medical research done on subjects deficient in vitamin E has shown that this nutrient helps prolong the life span of red blood cells.

For many American women, anemia can complicate a preexisting health-care condition. For example, anemia often accompanies thyroid disease, rheumatoid arthritis, and chronic kidney disease, as well as recurring or chronic infections. Anemia contributes to the fatigue and lack of energy that affect people suffering from these health problems. Anemia can also be caused by drugs that destroy or interfere with the utilization of the nutrients necessary for the health and maturation of the red blood cells. These drugs include oral contraceptives, alcohol, and anticonvulsive agents such as Dilantin.

In any case, the underlying causes of anemia must be reversed and corrected in order to reestablish healthy, normal red blood cells capable of carrying sufficient oxygen. When the anemia is corrected, the accompanying fatigue and lethargy will also be corrected.

The Nervous System

Depression

Depression is characterized as feeling so down or "blue" that these feelings interfere with daily life. One person in five in this country experiences symptoms of depression at some time. Thirty million people can expect to suffer from depression during their lifetimes, and 1.5 million people are currently undergoing treatment for this condition. Depression is twice as common in women as in men.

Depressed people suffer from a variety of symptoms that cause them to feel lethargic, fatigued, and unable to cope with other people and normal life activities. These symptoms include difficulty in concentrating and making decisions, and lack of self-esteem and self-confidence. Depressed women may suffer from a feeling of worthlessness and self-pity and may want to isolate themselves from other people to avoid social contact. Women with depression also display anxiety and irritability. They often suffer from eating problems (either overeating or undereating), insomnia, fatigue, digestive complaints, loss of sex drive, headaches, and backaches. Most dangerous to the women affected is that severe depression can lead to suicide attempts. Any threat of suicide in a depressed woman should be taken seriously and immediate medical care begun.

Many stressful life events can lead to depression, including death of a loved one, divorce, loss of a job, or even aging. Women who are experiencing low thyroid conditions, PMS, menopause, or the postpartum period are at higher risk of depression. Poor nutritional habits or the use of drugs and hormones (such as birth control pills and estrogen replacement therapy) can add to depression. Some women with depression are sensitive to the change of seasons. The shortness of the days and decreased light during the winter can trigger depression because the endocrine or glandular system may need more daylight to function optimally.

Women with depression may need a combination of antidepressive medication along with psychotherapy to combat the condition. Self-help techniques such as exercise, proper nutrition, and stress management can also be very helpful.

In summary, fatigue is an important symptom in many common health problems of women, including chronic fatigue syndrome, candida infections, allergies, PMS, menopause, hypothyroidism, anemia, and depression. Chapter 2 contains a workbook that will help you pinpoint any underlying physical problems that may be compounding your fatigue. It will also help you evaluate how your lifestyle habits may be contributing to increased tiredness.

Evaluating
Your Symptoms

2

The Chronic Fatigue Workbook

*T*his workbook section is a valuable tool to help you evaluate not only the symptoms and causes of your chronic fatigue, but also your lifestyle habits and how they contribute to your symptoms. If you take the time to fill out this section, you'll find it easier to recognize your weaknesses; then you can put together your personal treatment program from the chapters that follow.

First, fill out the checklist to evaluate your symptoms. I have included checklists on the diseases that commonly cause fatigue in women. Then, fill out the lifestyle habit evaluations; this will help you see which habit patterns are contributing to your chronic fatigue.

When you have completed the evaluation section, you will be ready to go on to the self-help chapters and begin your treatment program.

Evaluating Your Symptoms

Chronic Fatigue Syndrome

Chronic fatigue syndrome (CFS) affects 3 million people in the United States and 90 million people worldwide. For a true diagnosis of CFS, the symptoms must fulfill certain criteria.

Women with chronic fatigue must, with their physician's help, rule out any other disease that can mimic CFS symptoms. The fatigue must have lasted at least six months and be severely debilitating. The fatigue must also be accompanied by other characteristic symptoms (at least eight of those listed below in addition to fatigue itself). Check the symptoms that pertain to you.

	Yes	No
Fatigue that has persisted for six months or more and impairs daily activity by at least 50 percent	✕	—
Major symptoms developing over a few hours to a few days	—	—
Mild fever (less than 101.5°F oral), chills	—	✕
Sore throat, throat infections without pus	—	✕
Painful lymph nodes in the neck or armpits	—	✕
Unexplained generalized muscle weakness	✕	—
Muscle discomfort (myalgia)	—	✕
Prolonged (more than 24 hours) generalized fatigue following mild to moderate exercise	✕	—
Generalized headaches (different from any before this illness)	✕	—
Joint pains without swelling or redness	—	✕
Intolerance to light	✕	—
Blind spot in the visual field	—	✕
Irritability	—	✕
Forgetfulness, confusion, difficulty thinking, inability to concentrate	✕	—
Depression	✕	—
Sleep disturbance	—	✕

Candida Infections

Many women with a chronic candida problem suffer not only the common symptoms of chronic vaginal discharge and digestive upsets, but also fatigue and lethargy, as well as other symptoms. If candida seems to be your problem, check with your physician for a thorough evaluation. (The self-help suggestions in this book are also useful for the relief and prevention of candida.)

	Yes	No
Fatigue or lethargy	—	—
Depression	—	—
Poor memory, poor concentration	—	—
Persistent or recurrent vaginal discharge, itching, burning	—	—
Recurrent urinary burning, frequency	—	—
Abdominal bloating, pain, constipation, diarrhea, intestinal gas, mucus in bowel movements	—	—
Bad breath	—	—
Joint pain or swelling	—	—
Muscle aches or weakness	—	—
Numbness, tingling, burning	—	—
Headache	—	—
Nasal congestion, discharge, itching, postnasal drip	—	—
Skin rashes	—	—
Cough, tightness in chest, wheezing, shortness of breath	—	—
Poor visual activity, frequent tearing or burning of eyes	—	—
Menstrual dysfunction, cramps, premenstrual tension	—	—
Cravings for sugar, bread, or alcoholic beverages	—	—

Allergies

Women who have food or environmental allergies are often tired and lethargic if frequently exposed to the offending allergens. Allergens may also trigger uncomfortable symptoms in many different body systems. Check the symptoms that apply to you.

	Yes	No
Nasal congestion, sneezing, itching, postnasal drip		X
Redness, itching, or swelling of eyes; watery eyes, blurred vision, pain in eyes		X
Shortness of breath, wheezing, coughing, tightness or itching in throat		X
Popping or fullness in ears		X
Hives; itching, burning, or flushing of skin		X
Heartburn, indigestion, nausea, vomiting, diarrhea, itching or burning of rectum, abdominal pain or cramps		X
Frequent or urgent urination		X
Headaches	X	X
Sleepiness, slowness, sluggishness, dull feeling		X
Depression	X	X
Fatigue	X	
Tension, anxiety, hyperactivity, restlessness, excitability	X	
Inability to concentrate, difficulty in remembering words or names	X	

Premenstrual Syndrome

The most commonly experienced PMS symptoms are those that affect a woman's emotional well-being and energy level, including premenstrual fatigue. Other common symptoms include food cravings, bloating, headaches, and skin changes. Check the symptoms that pertain to your PMS pattern.

	Yes	No
Nervous tension		
Mood swings		
Irritability		
Anxiety		
Headache		

	Yes	No
Craving for sweets	___	___
Increased appetite	___	___
Pounding heart	___	___
Fatigue	___	___
Tremulousness	___	___
Depression	___	___
Forgetfulness	___	___
Crying	___	___
Sleeplessness	___	___
Weight gain	___	___
Swelling of extremities	___	___
Breast tenderness	___	___
Abdominal bloating	___	___
Oily skin	___	___
Oily hair	___	___
Pimples	___	___

Menopause

During the transition into menopause, women commonly experience many uncomfortable symptoms, including changes in mood and energy level. Many menopausal women have less energy and vitality than during their younger, reproductive years. Some women find that this affects their lifestyle and range of activities. If you have any of the menopausal symptoms listed below, follow the recommendations for relief in the self-help chapters of this book.

	Yes	No
Cessation of menstruation	___	___
Hot flashes	___	___
Night sweats	___	___
Vaginal dryness	___	___
Skin and hair dryness	___	___
Pain during sexual intercourse	___	___
Decrease in sex drive	___	___

	Yes	No
Increase in frequency of vaginal infections	—	—
Increase in urinary frequency	—	—
Loss of urine when sneezing or coughing	—	—
Increased frequency of urinary tract infections	—	—
Anxiety, irritability, mood swings	—	—
Depression, fatigue	—	—
Poor mental acuity and concentration	—	—
Insomnia	—	—
Weight gain	—	—
Poor muscle tone	—	—
Increased muscle weakness	—	—
Loss of muscle and bone mass	—	—

Hypothyroidism

Hypothyroidism is a common cause of tiredness in women. It increases with age and is far more common in women than in men (90 percent of the cases occur in women). If you suspect hypothyroidism on the basis of a positive response to the symptoms listed below, consult your physician; this can be easily diagnosed by blood testing. Follow the recommendations in the self-help chapters for optimal thyroid health.

	Yes	No
Hoarse voice	—	✓
Constipation	—	✓
Slowness of speech, thought, and movement	✓	—
Fatigue	✓	—
Intolerance to cold	—	✓
Thickening and scaling of skin	—	✓
Facial puffiness	—	✓
Delay of deep tendon reflexes	—	—
Low dietary iodine	—	—
Axillary (armpit) temperature below 97.8°F	—	—
Elevated cholesterol	—	—

Anemia and Heavy Menstrual Flow

The most common symptoms of anemia are listed below. The first five symptoms may occur in women with anemia caused by heavy menstrual bleeding. Check those that pertain to you. Some women have very few symptoms, while others have symptoms severe enough to affect their ability to function normally. The worse your symptoms, the more important it is to follow the self-help guidelines in this book.

	Yes	No
Fatigue	___	___
Dizziness	___	___
General weakness	___	___
Paleness	___	___
Profuse or extended menstrual bleeding	___	___
Loss of appetite	___	___
Brittle nails	___	___
Abdominal pain	___	___
Sore tongue	___	___
Yellowing of skin	___	___
Tingling in hands and feet	___	___
Loss of coordination	___	___
Diarrhea	___	___

Depression

Over 1.5 million people are treated for depression each year, including twice as many women as men. It is estimated that 30 million people suffer from depression during their lifetime. Check the symptoms that fit you. If your symptoms are severe, be sure to consult your physician. You can also follow the useful self-help suggestions in this book for chronic fatigue and depression.

	Yes	No
Fatigue	___	___
Feeling tearful, sad, "blue"	___	___
Tendency toward isolation, desire to be alone	___	___

	Yes	No
Difficulty in concentrating or making decisions	—	—
Poor mental acuity	—	—
Low self-esteem, little self-confidence	—	—
Self-dislike	—	—
Feeling of hopelessness	—	—
Suicidal thoughts and feelings	—	—
Difficulty sleeping	—	—
Overeating	—	—
Loss of appetite	—	—
Loss of sex drive	—	—
Digestive upsets	—	—
Headache	—	—
Backache	—	—

Evaluating Your Lifestyle Habits

The following charts allow you to evaluate the effect that your lifestyle habits have on your fatigue symptoms. Fill out the charts to see which areas of your life need to be modified to improve your energy level.

Eating Habits

Check the number of times you eat the following foods:

Food	Never	Once a month	Once a week	Twice a week +
Cow's milk			X	
Cow's cheese			X	
Butter				
Yogurt				X
Eggs	X			
Chocolate		X		X
Sugar				X

Food	Never	Once a month	Once a week	Twice a week +
Alcohol				X
Wheat bread				X
Wheat noodles				X
Wheat-based flour		X		
Pastries			X	
Added salt	X			
Bouillon				
Commercial salad dressing	X			
Catsup				X
Coffee	X			
Black tea	X			
Soft drinks				X
Hot dogs	X			
Ham		X		
Bacon				
Beef			X	
Lamb	X			X
Pork			X	

Foods in shaded area are "high stress" foods.

Food	Never	Once a month	Once a week	Twice a week +
Avocados				
Beans				
Beets				
Broccoli				
Brussels sprouts				
Cabbage				
Carrots				
Celery				
Collard greens				
Cucumbers				
Eggplant				

Food	Never	Once a month	Once a week	Twice a week +
Garlic				
Horseradish				
Kale				
Lettuce				
Mustard greens				
Okra				
Onions				
Parsnips				
Peas				
Potatoes				
Radishes				
Rutabagas				
Spinach				
Squash				
Sweet potatoes				
Tomatoes				
Turnips				
Yams				
Barley				
Brown rice				
Buckwheat				
Corn				
Millet				
Oatmeal				
Rye				
Raw flax seeds				
Raw pumpkin seeds				
Raw sesame seeds				
Raw sunflower seeds				
Raw almonds				
Raw filberts				
Raw pecans				

Food	Never	Once a month	Once a week	Twice a week +
Apples				
Bananas				
Berries				
Pears				
Seasonal fruits				
Corn oil				
Flax oil				
Olive oil				
Safflower oil				
Sesame oil				
Poultry				
Fish				

Key to Eating Habits

All foods in the shaded area are high-stress foods that are difficult to digest, stress the body's systems, and can increase the symptoms of chronic fatigue. If you eat many of these foods, or if you eat any of these foods frequently, your nutritional habits may be contributing significantly to your symptoms.

All foods in the unshaded area (from avocados through fish) are high-nutrient, low-stress foods that can be eaten on a regular basis by women who are already in a strong recovery from chronic fatigue. If your energy levels are approaching normal, you should include these foods frequently in your diet. Women who are just beginning a chronic fatigue self-help program will need a more restricted eating plan.

For further guidance on food selection, read Chapter 4, which explains the antifatigue diet, and Chapter 5, which offers specific menus, meal plans, and recipes. These recommendations and programs will help women just beginning a chronic fatigue recovery program as well as those who need a maintenance plan.

Exercise Habits

Check the number of times you do each of the following activities:

Activity	Never	Once a month	1 or 2x a week	3 x a week +
Walking				
Swimming				
Stretching				
Yoga				
Golf (with pull cart or caddy)				
Weight lifting (low stress)				
T'ai chi				
Slow dancing				

Key to Exercise Habits

Many women with chronic fatigue tend to lack physical endurance and stamina as well as feel a generalized tiredness. Even women accustomed to an active and vigorous exercise regimen may start to feel that any physical activity at all is just too difficult and may decide to stop exercising completely. This can have negative physiological effects on the body and worsen the fatigue symptoms. Although vigorous exercise may tire out a woman suffering from chronic fatigue and can be contraindicated, gentle exercise can provide the benefits of oxygenation, improved blood circulation, and muscle and joint flexibility. Exercise also helps to improve the mood as well as emotional and mental well-being—a welcome relief to many women with chronic fatigue. Select one or two of the less strenuous exercises given in the checklist and do them two or three times per week. Chapters 10 and 11 describe gentle exercise routines that you may find pleasant and easy to do.

Major Stress Evaluation

Checking many items in the first third of this scale indicates major life stress and a possible vulnerability to serious illness. In other words, the more items checked in the first third, the higher your stress quotient. *Do everything possible to manage your stress in a healthy way.* Eat the foods that provide a high-nutrient/low-stress diet, exercise on a regular basis, and learn the methods for managing stress given in the chapter on stress reduction and deep breathing.

If you check fewer items, you are probably at low risk of illness caused by stress. But because stresses too small to figure in this evaluation may also play a part in worsening your menstrual cramps, you would still benefit from practicing the methods outlined in the chapter on stress reduction. Stress management is very important in helping you to gain control over your own level of muscle tension.

Check the stressful events that apply to you.

___ Death of spouse or close family member
___ Divorce from spouse
___ Death of a close friend
___ Legal separation from spouse
___ Loss of job
___ Radical loss of financial security
___ Major personal injury or illness (gynecologic or other cause)
___ Future surgery for gynecologic or other illness
___ Beginning a new marriage
___ Foreclosure of mortgage or loan
___ Lawsuit lodged against you
___ Marriage reconciliation
___ Change in health of a family member
___ Major trouble with boss or co-workers
___ Increase in responsibility—job or home
___ Learning you are pregnant
___ Difficulties with your sexual abilities
___ Gaining a new family member
___ Change to a different job
___ Increase in number of marital arguments
___ New loan or mortgage of more than $100,000

___	Son or daughter leaving home
___	Major disagreement with in-laws or friends
___	Recognition for outstanding achievements
___	Spouse begins or stops work
___	Begin or end education
___	Undergo a change in living conditions
___	Revise or alter your personal habits
___	Change in work hours or conditions
___	Change of residence
___	Change your school or major in school
___	Alterations in your recreational activities
___	Change in church or club activities
___	Change in social activities
___	Change in sleeping habits
___	Change in number of family get-togethers
___	Diet or eating habits are changed
___	You go on vacation
___	The year-end holidays occur
___	You commit a minor violation of the law

Major life stress can have a significant impact on the symptoms of chronic fatigue as well as other health problems. It is helpful to assess your own level of stress to see how it may be impacting your health. One popular tool is the Holmes and Rahe Social Readjustment Rating Scale, first published in 1967. The scale above is adapted for women and identifies events that cause stress.

Daily Stress Evaluation

Check each item that seems to apply to you.

Work

___ **Too much responsibility.** You feel you have to push too hard to do your work. There are too many demands made of you. You feel pressured by all this responsibility. You worry about getting all your work done and doing it well.

_____ **Time urgency.** You worry about getting your work done on time. You always feel rushed, and feel there aren't enough hours in the day to complete your work.

_____ **Job instability.** You are concerned about losing your job. Your company is laying off employees. Your fellow employees are voicing insecurity and concern about job security.

_____ **Job performance.** You don't feel that you are working up to your maximum capability because of outside pressures or stress. You are unhappy with your own job performance and concerned about job security as a result.

_____ **Difficulty getting along with co-workers and boss.** Your boss is too picky and critical. Your boss demands too much. You must work closely with co-workers who are difficult to get along with.

_____ **Understimulation.** Work is boring. The lack of stimulation makes you tired. You wish you were somewhere else.

_____ **Uncomfortable physical plant.** Lights are too bright or too dim; noises are too loud. You're exposed to noxious fumes or chemicals. There is too much activity going on around you, making concentration difficult.

Spouse or Significant Other

_____ **Hostility.** Your relationship has too much negative emotion and drama. You are always upset and angry. There is not enough peace and quiet.

_____ **Not enough communication.** You and your significant other do not discuss feelings or issues enough. You both tend to hold in your feelings. You feel that an emotional bond is lacking between you.

_____ **Discrepancy in communication.** One person talks about feelings too much, the other person too little.

_____ **Affection.** You do not feel that you receive enough affection. There is not enough holding, touching, and loving in your relationship. Or, you are made uncomfortable by your partner's demands for affection.

_____ **Sexuality.** There's not enough sexual intimacy. You feel deprived by your partner. Or, your partner demands sexual relations too often. You feel pressured.

_____ **Children.** They make too much noise. They make too many demands on your time. They are hard to discipline.

_____ **Organization.** Home is poorly organized. It always seems messy; chores are half-finished.

_____ **Time.** You are inundated by too much to do in the home and never have enough time to get it all done.

_____ **Responsibility.** You need more help. There are too many demands on your time and energy.

Your Emotional State

_____ **Too much anxiety.** You worry too much about every little thing. You constantly worry about what can go wrong in your life.

_____ **Victimization.** Everyone is taking advantage of you or wants to hurt you.

_____ **Poor self-image.** You don't like yourself enough. You are always finding fault with yourself.

_____ **Too critical.** You are always finding fault with others. You always look at what is wrong with other people rather than seeing their virtues.

___ **Inability to relax.** You are always wound up. It is difficult for you to relax. You are tense and restless.

___ **Not enough self-renewal.** You don't play enough or take enough time off to relax and have fun. As a result, life isn't fun and enjoyable.

___ **Too angry.** Small life issues seem to upset you unduly. You find yourself becoming angry and irritable with your husband, children, or clients.

Key to Daily Stress Evaluation

This evaluation is very important for women with chronic fatigue. Not all stresses have a major impact in our lives, as do death, divorce, or personal injury. Most of us are exposed to a multitude of small life stresses on a daily basis. The effects of these stresses are cumulative and can be a major factor in triggering exhaustion. Becoming aware of them is the first step toward lessening their effect on your life. Methods for reducing stresses and helping your body deal with them are given in Chapter 7.

How Stress Affects Your Body

Each woman accumulates stress in a different way, tensing and contracting different sets of muscles in a pattern that is unique to her. High tension in your muscles worsens chronic fatigue. Muscle tension cuts off circulation and oxygenation to the affected parts of the body. Waste products of metabolism accumulate. This increase in waste products worsens your level of fatigue and lowers your energy and vitality. This evaluation should help you become aware of where you tend to carry stress.

Check the places where tension most commonly localizes in your body.

___ Low back
___ Pelvic area
___ Stomach muscles

___	Thighs and calves
___	Chest
___	Shoulders
___	Arms
___	Neck and throat
___	Headache
___	Grinding teeth
___	Eyestrain

It is important to be aware of where you store tension. When you feel tension building up in these areas, begin deep breathing exercises (Chapter 8) or use one of the stress reduction techniques given in Chapter 7. These techniques can help release muscle tension rapidly.

Finding
the Solution

3

Self-Help Program—
A Summary
Treatment Chart

*C*hapters 1 and 2 acquainted you with the causes and symptoms of chronic fatigue. You are now ready to put together your personal, antifatigue, self-help treatment program. All the techniques that you need are included in the chapters that follow; all have been very helpful to my patients. Treatment options include dietary and nutritional programs as well as very helpful routines for stress management, exercise, acupressure, and yoga.

The program is set up so that you can individualize a treatment plan for yourself. This chapter contains a summary chart that will help you put your program together. The chart lists the treatments that you can use for the relief of chronic fatigue; details are found in the following chapters.

You can use the summary chart in two ways. First, you can find your problem in the chart and turn directly to the treatments for the problem. I recommend that when beginning a program, you try all the therapies listed for your problem. You will probably find that some techniques make you feel better than others. Establish the regimen that works for you and practice it on a regular basis. Alternatively, you can read straight through the rest of the book to get a general overview of the various treatment techniques. Find the treatments you are interested in trying; then use the treatment chart for an overview and quick spot work. Either way of working with the book can bring you tremendous benefits. The most important thing is to follow your program on a regular basis. This will enable you to see improvement in your health and vitality very quickly—many women begin to feel better within a month or two.

Summary Treatment Chart for Chronic Fatigue

	Fatigue and Tiredness
Medication	nonspecific
Nutrition	The Antifatigue Diet
Vitamins, Minerals, Fatty Acids	Vitamin and mineral formula (page 115); emphasize vitamin B complex, vitamin C, potassium, magnesium, iron, zinc
Herbs	Peppermint, ginger, ginkgo biloba, licorice root, valerian root, passiflora, skullcap, hops, chamomile
Physical Exercise	Exercises 1, 2, 3
Breathing Exercises	Exercises 1, 2, 3, 4, 5, 6, 7, 8, 9
Stress	Exercises 1, 2, 3, 4, 5, 6, 7, 8, 9
Yoga	Exercises 1, 2, 3, 4, 5, 6, 7, 8, 9
Acupressure	Exercises 1, 2, 3, 4, 5, 6, 7, 8, 9

Summary Treatment Chart for Chronic Fatigue

	Chronic Fatigue Syndrome	Candida Infections
Medication	Tagamet, Zantac, dox-epin, Prozac, Elavil, gamma globulin, transfer factor, alpha interferon	Nystatin, Nizoral, Diflucan
Nutrition	The Antifatigue Diet	The Antifatigue Diet
Vitamins, Minerals, Fatty Acids	Emphasize vitamin A, vitamin B complex, phosphatidyl-choline, vitamin C, quercetin, magnesium, calcium, iron, chromium	Emphasize vitamin A, vitamin B complex, vitamin C, vitamin E, magnesium, iron, zinc, essential fatty acids, caprylic acid
Herbs	Peppermint, aloe vera, ginger, ginkgo biloba, licorice root, garlic, echinacea, goldenseal, valerian root, passi-flora, skullcap, hops, chamomile	Pau d'arco, garlic, echinacea, goldenseal
Physical Exercise	Exercises 1, 2, 3	Exercises 1, 2, 3
Breathing Exercises	Exercises 1, 2, 3, 4, 5, 6, 7, 8, 9	Exercises 1, 2, 3, 4, 5, 6, 7, 8, 9
Stress	Exercises 1, 2, 3, 4, 5, 6, 7, 8, 9	Exercises 1, 2, 3, 4, 5, 6, 7, 8, 9
Yoga	Exercises 1, 2, 3, 4, 5, 6*, 7*, 8*, 9	Exercises 1, 2, 3, 4, 5, 6*, 7*, 8*, 9
Acupressure	Exercises 1*, 2, 3, 4, 5*	Exercises 1*, 2, 3, 4, 5*

The starred (*) exercises are particularly effective for the problems listed.

	Allergies	Premenstrual Syndrome (PMS)
Medication	Antihistamines, decongestants	Progesterone, birth control pills, diuretics, antidepressants
Nutrition	The Antifatigue Diet	The Antifatigue Diet
Vitamins, Minerals, Fatty Acids	Emphasize vitamin A, vitamin B_{12}, vitamin C, bioflavonoids, quercetin, bromelain, essential fatty acids	Emphasize vitamin B complex (especially B_6), magnesium, potassium, iodine, essential fatty acids
Herbs	Ginger, licorice root	Chaste tree berry, cramp bark, wild yam, ginger, valerian root, skullcap, hops, passiflora, chamomile
Physical Exercise	Exercises 1, 2, 3	Exercises 1, 2, 3
Breathing Exercises	Exercises 1, 2, 3, 4, 5, 6, 7, 8, 9	Exercises 1, 2, 3, 4, 5, 6, 7, 8, 9
Stress	Exercises 1, 2, 3, 4, 5, 6, 7, 8, 9	Exercises 1, 2, 3, 4, 5, 6, 7, 8, 9
Yoga	Exercises 1, 2, 3, 4, 5, 6*, 7*, 8*, 9	Exercises 1, 2, 3, 4, 5*, 6*, 7, 8, 9
Acupressure	Exercises 1*, 2, 3, 4, 5*	Exercises 1, 2, 3*, 4, 6*

The starred (*) exercises are particularly effective for the problems listed.

Summary Treatment Chart for Chronic Fatigue

	Menopause	Low Thyroid Function (Hypothyroidism)
Medication	Estrogen, progestins, antidepressants, tranquilizers	Thyroid replacement therapy
Nutrition	The Antifatigue Diet	The Antifatigue Diet
Vitamins, Minerals, Fatty Acids	Emphasize vitamin E, vitamin C, bioflavonoids, potassium, magnesium, calcium, chromium, manganese, iodine, essential fatty acids	Emphasize iodine, vitamin C, choline, vitamin B_6, L-tyrosine
Herbs	Fennel, anise, red clover, licorice, wild yam, Oregon grape root, wild cherry bark, sarsaparilla, ginger, ginkgo biloba, valerian root, passiflora, skullcap, hops, chamomile	Kelp, dulse
Physical Exercise	Exercises 1, 2, 3	Exercises 1, 2, 3
Breathing Exercises	Exercises 1, 2, 3, 4, 5, 6, 7, 8, 9	Exercises 1, 2, 3, 4, 5, 6, 7, 8, 9
Stress	Exercises 1, 2, 3, 4, 5, 6, 7, 8, 9	Exercises 1, 2, 3, 4, 5, 6, 7, 8, 9
Yoga	Exercises 1, 2, 3, 4, 5*, 6*, 7, 8, 9	Exercises 1*, 2*, 3*, 4, 5, 6, 7, 8, 9
Acupressure	Exercises 1, 2, 3*, 4, 5, 6*	Exercises 1, 2, 3, 4, 7*, 8*

The starred (*) exercises are particularly effective for the problems listed.

Summary Treatment Chart for Chronic Fatigue

	Anemia	Depression
Medication	Thyroid replacement therapy, anti-infectious agents, medications for specific chronic disease problems	Antidepressants
Nutrition	The Antifatigue Diet	The Antifatigue Diet
Vitamins, Minerals, Fatty Acids	Emphasize iron, folic acid, vitamin B_{12}, vitamin B_6, vitamin C, vitamin E	Emphasize vitamin B complex, vitamin C, potassium, magnesium, calcium, essential fatty acids, phenylalanine, tryptophan, L-tyrosine
Herbs	Shepherd's purse, pau d'arco, yellow dock, goldenseal, hawthorn berry, grape skins, cherry, bilberry, Oregon grape root	Ginger, ginkgo biloba, licorice root, peppermint, Siberian ginseng, oat straw
Physical Exercise	Exercises 1, 2, 3	Exercises 1, 2, 3
Breathing Exercises	Exercises 1, 2, 3, 4, 5, 6, 7, 8, 9	Exercises 1, 2, 3, 4, 5, 6, 7, 8, 9
Stress	Exercises 1, 2, 3, 4, 5, 6, 7, 8, 9	Exercises 1, 2, 3, 4, 5, 6, 7, 8, 9
Yoga	Exercises 1*, 2*, 3,* 4, 5, 6*, 7*, 8*, 9	Exercises 1*, 2*, 3, 4, 5, 6, 7, 8, 9*
Acupressure	Exercises 1, 2, 3, 4, 9*	Exercises 1, 2*, 3, 4, 5*, 6*

The starred (*) exercises are particularly effective for the problems listed.

4

Dietary Principles for Relief of Chronic Fatigue

$\mathcal{D}$iet plays a major role in creating or relieving the symptoms of chronic fatigue. I have found during my years of practice that if women ignore the importance of nutrition in their antifatigue program, they have great difficulty getting entirely well. Women recovering from fatigue need to follow a low-stress diet that is high in nutritional value. Although food provides the energy to fuel the hundreds of thousands of chemical reactions that occur continuously, some foods are not easily used or well tolerated by the body.

In this chapter, I list and discuss in detail the foods that worsen chronic fatigue and should be avoided. The list may surprise you, because it contains not only processed "junk food," but also foods that are considered staples of the American diet. Many women with chronic fatigue unwittingly eat a diet that worsens their symptoms. I also discuss foods that can improve and enhance your energy level, as well as help you make the transition into healthier eating habits. This information is based on extensive work with women who have suffered from fatigue and noted significant relief of their symptoms when following this program.

Foods to Avoid

It is important to eliminate all foods that diminish your energy reserves. These include foods that are difficult to digest, as well as foods that are toxic to and damaging to the body. The process of digestion itself takes a lot of energy. Digestion must occur before the body can extract energy from the foods you eat. Proteins must be broken down into amino acids, complex carbohydrates into simple sugars, and fats into fatty acids. For these breakdowns to occur, food is chemically acted upon by stomach acid, hormones, pancreatic enzymes, and fat emulsifiers, as well as by the mechanical process that propels food through the entire length of the digestive tract. Once the food is broken down, it must then be absorbed from the digestive tract and taken into the blood. From there, the food particles circulate to cells throughout the body. At this cellular level, the energy contained in the food is finally captured to fuel the body's many chemical and physiological reactions.

This entire process requires a great deal of work. The body needs a lot of reserve energy to produce the chemicals involved in the digestive process. As a result, women with chronic fatigue need to eat foods that require the least amount of work to break down, yet still contain the highest level of nutrients.

Unfortunately, many of the most commonly eaten foods in our society are hard to digest. These include foods that are high in saturated fats, sugars, and animal protein. The long list includes pizza, steaks, bacon, cheeseburgers, french fries, doughnuts, ice cream, hot dogs, chocolate, and many other processed and high-stress foods. For example, the body must work hard to digest a meal of thick steak, french fries, buttered bread, wine, and a chocolate dessert. This meal is laden with saturated fats, red meat protein, and sugar. On finishing this meal, a woman will feel overly full and more tired than before she started eating. In contrast, a light meal of bean soup, mixed green salad, and baked potato is full of vitamins, minerals, carbohydrates, and easy-to-digest vegetable-based protein. It is also low in fat and sugar. These foods are much more likely to leave you feeling energized and comfortable.

Other foods stress the body through their toxicity. There are many mechanisms by which a food can increase fatigue. Some foods have a toxic effect that damages the cells and affects their ability to function. One good example is alcohol, which is particularly toxic to the liver, brain, and nervous system. Some foods, such as alcohol and sugar, promote the growth of pathological organisms like candida, which can worsen fatigue. Many food additives and preservatives can cause an allergic or toxic reaction in susceptible women. The following foods should be avoided by women with chronic fatigue, either because they are difficult to digest or because of their toxic effects on the body.

Caffeine. Coffee, black tea, soft drinks, and chocolate—all these foods contain caffeine, an unhealthy stimulant used to increase energy levels and alertness and decrease fatigue. Many women with chronic fatigue mistakenly use caffeine as a pick-me-up to help them get through the day's tasks. Unfortunately, caffeine can actually worsen fatigue. Caffeine used in excess increases anxiety, irritability, and mood swings. Even small amounts can cause susceptible women to become jittery. After the initial pick-up, women with chronic fatigue find that caffeine intake makes them more tired than before; it depletes energy and physical reserves by stressing the nervous system and exhausting the adrenal glands. Caffeine also depletes the body's stores of B-complex vitamins and essential minerals, which are important in the chemical reactions that convert food to usable energy. Deficiency of these nutrients worsens fatigue. Depletion of B-complex vitamins also interferes with carbohydrate metabolism and healthy liver function, which helps to regulate estrogen levels. An imbalance in estrogen and progesterone can worsen fatigue and mood swings in women with symptoms of PMS or menopause. Many menopausal women also complain that caffeine increases the frequency of hot flashes. Coffee, black tea, chocolate, and soft drinks all act to inhibit iron absorption, thus worsening anemia.

Sugar. Like caffeine, sugar depletes the body's B-complex vitamins and minerals, thereby increasing nervous tension, anxiety, and irritability. Excessive glucose intake disrupts carbohydrate metabolism directly by overworking the pancreas and adrenal glands, worsening the symptoms of fatigue and hypoglycemia. Too much sugar also intensifies fatigue by causing vasoconstriction (the narrowing of the diameter of blood vessels) and putting stress on the nervous system. Candida feeds on sugar, so overindulging in this high-stress food worsens chronic candida infections.

Unfortunately, sugar addiction is common in our society among people of all ages. Many people use sweet foods as a way to deal with their frustrations and other upsets. As a result, most Americans eat too much sugar—the average American eats 120 pounds per year. Many convenience foods, including salad dressing, catsup, and relish, contain high levels of both sugar and salt. Sugar is the main ingredient in soft drinks and in desserts such as candies, cookies, cakes, and ice cream. Highly sugared foods also lead to tooth loss through tooth decay and gum disease. Of even greater significance is the fact that excess sugar intake can worsen diabetes.

In summary, sugar stresses many bodily systems, worsens your health, and intensifies fatigue. Try to satisfy your sweet tooth instead with healthier foods, such as fruit or grain-based desserts like oatmeal cookies sweetened with fruit or honey. You will find that small amounts of these foods can satisfy your cravings. Instead of disrupting your mood and energy level, they actually have a healthful and balancing effect.

Alcohol. Women with chronic fatigue should avoid alcohol entirely. Alcohol has a sedative effect. Many women with fatigue caused by PMS, menopause, CFS, candida, or allergies find that their bodies do not tolerate even small amounts of alcohol. Besides worsening fatigue and making women feel sleepy, alcohol affects mental faculties. Women with chronic fatigue often complain that alcohol makes them feel "spacey," "ungrounded," and unable to concentrate or process information efficiently. Besides being directly toxic to the brain and nervous system, alcohol depletes the body's B-complex vitamins and minerals such as magnesium by disrupting carbohydrate metabolism. In women with PMS, depletion of magnesium and B-complex vitamins can also intensify menstrual fatigue and mood swings.

Candida thrive not only on sugar, but also on alcohol—so alcohol promotes their growth in the body. Women with candida-related fatigue need to avoid alcohol entirely. Many women with allergies are sensitive to the yeasts in the alcohol, which worsen their allergic symptoms. Alcohol is toxic to the liver and can affect the liver's ability to metabolize hormones efficiently. Excessive alcohol intake has been associated with lack of ovulation and elevated estrogen levels, which can trigger fibroid growth and heavy bleeding, particularly in women who are in transition into menopause and have a progesterone deficiency.

When used carefully—not exceeding 4 ounces of wine per day, 10 ounces of beer, or 1 ounce of hard liquor—alcohol can have a delightfully relaxing effect in women who have normal energy levels. It can make us more sociable and enhance the taste of food. For optimal health, however, I recommend that women with chronic fatigue use alcohol only very rarely. Women who are particularly susceptible to the negative effects of alcohol shouldn't drink at all. If you entertain a great deal and enjoy social drinking, try nonalcoholic beverages. A nonalcoholic cocktail, such as mineral water with twist of lime or lemon or a dash of bitters, is a good substitute. Near beer is a nonalcoholic beer substitute that tastes quite good. Light wine and beer have a lower alcohol content than hard liquor, liqueurs, and regular wine.

Dairy Products. For women with chronic fatigue, dairy products are high-stress foods. This always surprises women, because dairy products have traditionally been touted as one of the four basic food groups, and many women use them as staples in their diet, eating large amounts of cheese, yogurt, milk, and cottage cheese. Yet dairy products are extremely difficult for the body to digest; they can worsen fatigue because the body must use so much energy to break them down before they can be absorbed, assimilated, and finally utilized. All parts of dairy products are difficult to digest—the fat, the protein, and the milk sugar. Digesting dairy products demands hydrochloric acids, enzymes, and fat emulsifiers, which a fatigued woman may not produce in sufficient quantities.

Many women are specifically allergic to dairy products, and dairy products intensify allergy symptoms in general. Besides fatigue, users of dairy products often complain of allergy-based nasal congestion, sinus swelling, and postnasal drip. They can also suffer from digestive problems such as bloating, gas, and bowel changes, which intensify with menstruation. This intolerance to dairy products can hamper the absorption and assimilation of the calcium they contain. Also, clinical studies have shown that dairy products decrease iron absorption in anemic women.

Dairy products have many other unhealthy effects on a woman's body. The tryptophan in milk has a sedative effect that increases fatigue, a real problem for some women the first day or two of their periods, as well as for women suffering from depression. Menopausal women, who suffer from fatigue caused by the decline in hormonal levels, can also be sensitive to the tryptophan levels in dairy products. Besides worsening fatigue symptoms, the saturated fats in dairy products put women at higher risk of heart disease and cancer of the breast, uterus, and ovaries. Women on a high-fat diet also tend to accumulate excess weight more easily.

Women who have depended on dairy products for their calcium intake naturally wonder what alternative sources they should use. Women concerned about calcium intake can turn to many other good dietary sources of this essential nutrient, including beans, peas, soybeans, sesame seeds, soup stock made from chicken or fish bones, and green leafy vegetables. For food preparation, soy milk, potato milk, and nut milk are excellent substitutes. These nondairy milks are readily available at health food stores. You can also use a supplement containing calcium, magnesium, and vitamin D to make sure your intake is sufficient.

Red Meats and Poultry. Like dairy products, meat tends to increase fatigue because it is difficult for the body to digest. Because of the extremely tough protein found in meat, as well as its high content of saturated fats, the body must work hard to reduce the protein to amino acids and the saturated fats to fatty acids. Many women with chronic fatigue feel exhausted after a heavy meal of meat. Besides the difficulty of digesting meat and the energy expended in the process, meat intake can also worsen fatigue in other ways. The body uses the fatty acids found in meat (and dairy products) to produce a group of hormones called the series-two prostaglandins. These hormones, found in tissues throughout the body, have negative health effects. They cause contraction of muscles and blood vessels and thereby worsen cramps, PMS, high blood pressure, and irritable bowel syndrome. These hormones also put stress on the immune function and trigger inflammation. As a result, they can worsen infections of all types, decrease resistance, and trigger allergy symptoms. Eating meat with high saturated fat content as a major part of the diet, like eating dairy products, puts women at risk of heart disease, breast cancer, and cancer of the reproductive tract, as well as obesity. Women with chronic fatigue should sharply curtail such consumption.

Instead of eating meat, obtain your protein from vegetable sources, such as legumes, starches, raw seeds, and grains. You may eat fish occasionally, too. Fish has the added benefit of containing high levels of essential fatty acids, which improve vitality.

Wheat and Other Gluten-Containing Grains. Women with chronic fatigue have difficulty digesting wheat. The protein in wheat, called gluten, is highly allergenic and difficult for the body to break down, absorb, and assimilate. No matter what the cause of your chronic fatigue, if the symptoms are severe, you should probably eliminate wheat from your diet, at least in the early stages of recovery.

Women with wheat intolerance are prone to fatigue, depression, bloating, intestinal gas, and bowel changes. Wheat consumption by depressed women who are nutritionally sensitive can worsen emotional symptoms. I have seen wheat worsen fatigue in my PMS patients during the week or two before the onset of menses. Many menopausal women tolerate wheat poorly because their digestive tracts are beginning to show the wear and tear of aging and don't produce enough enzymes to handle wheat easily. Women with allergies often find that wheat intensifies nasal and sinus congestion as well as fatigue. I also find that women with poor resistance and a tendency toward infections may need to eliminate wheat to boost their immune function. Since wheat is leavened with yeast, it should be also avoided by women with candida infections.

Oats and rye, which also contain gluten, should be eliminated along with wheat. Many allergic and severely fatigued women don't even handle corn or rice well. Although these do not contain gluten, most women use them so frequently that they build up an intolerance during times of fatigue.

I have found over the years that the least stressful grain for fatigued women is buckwheat. This is probably because it is not commonly eaten in our society. Also, it is not in the same plant family as wheat and other grains. As women with fatigue start to regain their vitality and become more energetic, they can add rice and corn back into the diet, still eliminating wheat, oats, and rye until their recovery is complete.

Salt.   Although salt does not specifically worsen chronic fatigue, women should watch their salt intake carefully and avoid excessive intake for optimal health and well-being. Too much salt in the diet can cause many physical symptoms. It can worsen bloating and fluid retention, thereby contributing to the symptoms of PMS and menstrual cramps. Too much salt intake can also worsen high blood pressure and is a risk factor in the development of osteoporosis in menopausal women. Unfortunately, most processed foods contain large amounts of salt. Frozen and canned foods are often loaded with salt. In fact, one frozen-food entree can contribute as much as one-half teaspoon of salt to your daily intake. Large amounts of salt are also commonly found in the American diet as table salt (sodium chloride), MSG (monosodium glutamate), and a variety of food additives. Fast foods such as hamburgers, hot dogs, french fries, pizza, and tacos are loaded with salt and saturated fats. Common processed foods such as soups, potato chips, cheese, olives, salad dressings, and catsup (to name only a few) are also very high in salt. To make matters worse, many people use too much salt while cooking and seasoning their meals.

For women of all ages, I recommend eliminating added salt in your meals. For flavor, use seasonings such as garlic, herbs, spices, and lemon juice. Avoid processed foods that are high in salt, including canned foods, olives, pickles, potato chips, tortilla chips, catsup, and salad dressings. Learn to read labels and look for the word *sodium* (salt). If it appears high on the list of ingredients, don't buy the product. Many items in health food stores are labeled "no salt added." Some supermarkets offer "no added salt" foods in their diet or health food sections.

Foods to Avoid with Chronic Fatigue
Coffee

Tea (non-herbal)

Chocolate

Cola drinks

Sugar

Alcohol

Dairy products

Red meat, poultry

Fried and fatty foods

Convenience foods

Wheat, oats, rye

Salt

Foods That Help Relieve Chronic Fatigue

I have always worked with my chronic fatigue patients to design a dietary program that gives them the best quality nutrients. The foods that a fatigued woman eats should leave her feeling as good as, if not better than, she felt before the meal. These foods should also support and accelerate the healing process of the illness that underlies the fatigue. To achieve these goals means initially limiting your diet to low-stress foods. As your fatigue symptoms diminish, you can eat a wider range of foods. I help my patients develop an awareness of how their food selections affect their energy levels. If a particular food lowers your energy level each time you eat it, you should eliminate it.

I have found that certain groups of foods are tolerated by nearly everyone, even women who are severely fatigued. These foods include most vegetables, certain fruits, starches, a few grain alternatives such as buckwheat, and a few types of seeds and nuts. Initially, these should be your core food selection. As you feel better, you can add more fruits, grains, oils, fish, and poultry.

The only major exception is severely fatigued women who are suffering from anemia. Anemic women have very specific nutritional needs. To rebuild their stores of blood cells, women with anemia should read the nutritional chapters of my book *Anemia & Heavy Menstrual Flow* for more specific dietary guidelines. Otherwise, women with chronic fatigue need to have an easily digestible, stress-free diet. In this section I discuss in detail the benefits of the foods that I recommend for fatigue.

Vegetables. These are outstanding foods for the relief of chronic fatigue. Many vegetables are high in calcium, magnesium, and potassium—important minerals that help improve stamina, endurance, and vitality. Both magnesium and potassium, used in supplemental form in clinical studies, have been shown to increase energy levels dramatically. For women with chronic fatigue who suffer from tension and anxiety, the essential minerals in vegetables have a relaxant effect, relieving muscular tension and calming the emotions, too. Both calcium and magnesium act as natural tranquilizers, a real benefit for women suffering from stress and upset. The potassium content of vegetables helps relieve the congestive symptoms of PMS by reducing fluid retention and bloating. Some of the best sources for these minerals include Swiss chard, spinach, broccoli, beet greens, mustard greens, and kale. These vegetables are also high in iron, which can help relieve anemia and menstrual cramps.

Many vegetables are high in vitamin C, which helps increase capillary permeability and facilitate the flow of essential nutrients throughout the body, as well as the flow of waste products out. Vitamin C is also an important antistress vitamin because it is needed for healthy adrenal hormone production (the adrenal glands help us deal with stress). This is particularly important for women with chronic fatigue caused by infections, allergies, emotional upset, or stress from other origins. Vitamin C is also important for immune function and wound healing. Its anti-infectious properties may help reduce the tendency toward respiratory, bladder, and vaginal infections. Vegetables high in vitamin C include brussels sprouts, broccoli, cauliflower, kale, peppers, parsley, peas, tomatoes, and potatoes.

Carrots, spinach, squash, turnip greens, collards, parsley, green onions, and kale are among the vegetables highest in vitamin A. Vitamin A is important for women with chronic fatigue whose resistance is low and who are thus prone to infections. Vitamin A strengthens the cell walls and protects the mucous membranes. This helps protect you from respiratory disease as well as allergic episodes. Vitamin A deficiency has been linked to fatigue as well as night blindness, skin aging, loss of smell, loss of appetite, and softening of bones and teeth. Luckily, it is easy to get an abundance of vitamin A in the diet from vegetables.

Vegetables are composed primarily of water and carbohydrates. Because they contain very little protein and fat, they tend to be easy to digest. However, in the early stages of recovery, women with chronic fatigue may find that they more easily digest cooked vegetables. Cooking serves to break down the fiber in the vegetables and render it softer in texture, making less work for the body in the digestion process. Steaming is the best cooking method, because it preserves the essential nutrients. Some women with extreme fatigue may even want to puree their vegetables in a blender. As you begin to recover your energy, I recommend adding raw foods such as salads, juices, and raw vegetables to your meals for more texture and variety.

Fruits. Fruits also contain a wide range of nutrients that can relieve chronic fatigue. Like many vegetables, fruits are an excellent source of vitamin C, which is important for healthy blood vessels and blood circulation throughout the body, as well as for its antistress and immune-stimulant properties. Almost all fruits contain some vitamin C, the best sources being berries and melons. These fruits are also good sources of bioflavonoids, another essential nutrient that affects blood vessel strength and permeability. Bioflavonoids also have an anti-inflammatory effect, important to women with allergies, menstrual cramps, or arthritis. Bioflavonoids are supportive of the female reproductive tract and can improve mood and increase energy levels in women with PMS or menopausal symptoms. Although citrus fruits (oranges, grapefruits) are excellent sources of bioflavonoids and vitamin C, they are highly acidic and difficult for many women with chronic fatigue to digest; therefore, such women should avoid them in the early stages of treatment.

Certain fruits—including raisins, blackberries, and bananas— are excellent sources of calcium and magnesium; you can eat them often. Raisins and bananas are also exceptional sources of potassium, good for women with chronic fatigue and bloating. All fruits, in fact, are excellent sources of potassium.

Eat fruits whole to benefit from their high fiber content, which helps prevent constipation and other digestive irregularities. For snacks and desserts, fresh fruits are excellent substitutes for cookies, candies, cakes, and other foods high in refined sugar. Although fruit is high in sugar, its high fiber content helps slow down absorption of the sugar into the blood circulation and thereby helps stabilize the blood sugar level. I recommend, however, that women with chronic fatigue do not consume fruit juices. Fruit juice does not contain the bulk or fiber of the whole fruit. As a result, it acts more like table sugar and can destabilize your blood sugar level dramatically when used to excess. This can exacerbate fatigue and mood swings.

Starches. Potatoes, sweet potatoes, and yams are soft, well-tolerated carbohydrates that provide an additional source of easy-to-digest protein for women with chronic fatigue. You can steam, mash, bake, and eat them alone, or include them in other low-stress dishes and casseroles. Starches combine very well with a variety of vegetables and can form the basis of delicious, low-stress meals. You can also combine them with lentils or split peas in soup.

Potatoes, especially sweet potatoes, are an exceptional source of vitamin A, so they can help boost resistance in women prone to infections and allergies. Potatoes and yams are also good sources of vitamin C and several of the B vitamins that reduce fatigue and help women handle stress better.

Legumes. Beans and peas are excellent sources of energy-building calcium, magnesium, and potassium. I highly recommend their use in a diet to combat fatigue. However, because they also contain high levels of protein, women with severe fatigue may find them difficult to digest at first. For easier digestibility, I recommend beginning with green beans, green peas, split peas, lentils, lima beans, fresh sprouts, and possibly tofu (if you handle soy products well). As your energy level improves, add such delicious legumes as black beans, pinto beans, kidney beans, and chickpeas. These foods are high in iron and tend to be good sources of copper and zinc. Legumes are very high in vitamin B complex and vitamin B_6, necessary nutrients for the relief and prevention of menstrual fatigue and cramps. They are also excellent sources of protein and, when eaten with grains, provide all the essential amino acids. (Good examples of low-stress grain and legume combinations include meals of beans and buckwheat, or corn bread and split pea soup.) Legumes provide an excellent, easily utilized source of protein and can be substituted for meat at many meals.

Legumes are an excellent source of fiber that can help normalize bowel function. They digest slowly and can help to regulate the blood sugar level, a trait they share with whole grains. As a result, legumes are an excellent food for women with diabetes or blood sugar imbalances. Some women find that gas is a problem when they eat beans. You can minimize gas by taking digestive enzymes and eating beans in small quantities.

Whole Grains. Although you should eliminate most grains from your diet (especially wheat and other gluten-containing grains) when first starting an antifatigue program, you may be able to use a few grainlike alternatives in the initial stages. These include buckwheat and more exotic grain alternatives, such as quinoa and amaranth. They do not actually belong in the grain family, yet pasta, cereals, and other foods made from these grain alternatives can be purchased in health food stores. You may find that they don't cause the fatigue symptoms that commonly used grains like wheat, oats, and rye often trigger.

I usually exclude corn and rice from the diet of severely fatigued women. As symptoms begin to improve, you can try adding these foods back into your diet. I suggest adding them back slowly and rotating them with the grain alternatives so you don't overdose your body on any one grain. This helps prevent allergic reactions and fatigue. Besides eating corn and rice as grains, you can find pasta and noodles, as well as flour for baking, made from these grains. Use corn tortillas instead of those made of wheat.

Seeds and Nuts. Seeds and nuts are the best sources of the two essential fatty acids, linoleic acid and linolenic acid. These fatty acids provide the raw materials your body needs to produce the beneficial prostaglandin hormones. Adequate levels of essential fatty acids in your diet are very important in preventing symptoms of PMS, menopause, emotional upsets, allergies, and lowered resistance. The best sources of both fatty acids are raw flax and pumpkin seeds. Other seeds, such as sesame and sunflower seeds, are excellent sources of linoleic acid alone. Seeds and nuts are also excellent sources of the B-complex vitamins and vitamin E, both of which are important antistress factors for women with fatigue. These nutrients also help regulate hormonal balance and relieve PMS and menopausal symptoms.

Like vegetables, seeds and nuts are very high in the essential minerals such as magnesium, calcium, and potassium needed by women with fatigue. Particularly beneficial are sesame seeds, sunflower seeds, pistachios, pecans, and almonds; however, they are very high in calories and can be difficult to digest. Therefore, seeds and nuts should be eaten only in small amounts or avoided entirely by women with severe fatigue until their symptoms begin to improve. Women with fatigue may find that they can tolerate fresh flax seed oil, and their symptoms may even improve with its continued dietary use. Flax seed oil is one of the best sources of the essential fatty acids needed for production of the beneficial prostaglandin hormones.

The oils in seeds and nuts are very perishable, so avoid exposing them to light, heat, and oxygen. Try to eat them raw, and shell them yourself. Eating them raw and unsalted gives you the benefit of their essential fatty acids (beneficial for skin and hair) and you'll also avoid the negative effects of too much salt. If you buy them already shelled, refrigerate them so their oils don't become rancid. Seeds and nuts make a wonderful garnish on salads, vegetable dishes, and casseroles. As your energy level improves, you can also eat them as a main source of protein with snacks and light meals.

Meat, Poultry, and Fish. I generally recommend eating meat only in small quantities or avoiding it altogether if you have severe chronic fatigue, because red meats like beef, pork, and lamb, as well as poultry, contain saturated fats and hard-to-digest protein. If you do want to eat meat, your best choice is fish. Unlike other meat, fish contains linolenic acid, one of the beneficial fatty acids that help relax tense muscles, a major cause of fatigue in women. Fish is also an excellent source of minerals, especially iodine and potassium. Particularly good fish for women with chronic fatigue are salmon, tuna, mackerel, and trout.

If you do include meat in your antifatigue program, I recommend using it in very small amounts (3 ounces or less per day). Most Americans eat much more protein than is healthy. Excessive amounts of protein are difficult to digest and stress the kidneys. All meats, except fish, are prime sources of unhealthy saturated fats, which put you at higher risk of heart disease and cancer. Instead of using meat as your only source of protein, I recommend increasing your intake of grains, beans, raw seeds, and nuts, which contain not only protein but also many other important nutrients. For many years I have recommended that my patients use meat more as a garnish and a flavoring for casseroles, stir-fries, and soups. I also recommend buying meat from organic, range-fed animals, as their exposure to pesticides, antibiotics, and hormones has been reduced. If you find meat difficult to digest, you may be deficient in hydrochloric acid. Try taking a small amount of hydrochloric acid with every meat-containing meal to see if your digestion improves.

How to Change to a Healthier Diet

Please don't feel that you need to make all your dietary changes at once. To do so is stressful for anyone, and particularly for a woman with chronic fatigue. Make all nutritional changes gradually and at a pace that feels comfortable to you. Some of my patients eliminate all high-stress foods immediately, while others do it slowly over time. You may want to start by eliminating one or two high-stress foods from your diet. After you become comfortable with these initial changes, review the lists of foods to eliminate and foods to emphasize in your diet. Then choose several more foods that you are willing to drop from your menus and try several new ones.

Occasionally, women find that they actually feel worse when they first eliminate high-stress foods such as chocolate, alcohol, coffee, or sugar. This reaction can last a few days or up to several weeks. Your fatigue may actually worsen or you may be irritable, jittery, and suffer from headaches or nasal congestion. You may also crave the foods that you've eliminated. Generally, these are symptoms of withdrawal from foods to which you've actually been addicted. Once the critical period passes, you will begin to feel much better. I generally recommend that women follow the elimination diet carefully throughout their entire recovery from fatigue. In the next chapter you will find meal plans and recipes to make the process easier.

Once you have regained your energy, you may want to reintroduce some of the high-stress foods into your diet. I would caution you to do it slowly, and never to excess. Chocolate, alcohol, sugar, colas, coffee, dairy products, and red meat are foods that should be limited in anyone's diet for optimal health and well-being. As long as you follow the general principles proposed in this chapter, your diet should help you recover and maintain your energy and vitality.

5

Menus,
Meal Plans,
& Recipes

CHIVES

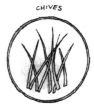

$\mathcal{M}$eal planning is particularly important for women with chronic fatigue. When your energy reserves are low, even the occasional rich meal laden with fats and sugar, eaten at a restaurant or a party, can exhaust you. Frequent meals of high-stress foods can worsen your symptoms significantly and retard your recovery. Women with chronic fatigue need meals high in nutrient content, yet easy to digest. In addition, meals should be quick and easy to prepare, so that food preparation doesn't exhaust your limited energy reserves.

To achieve these goals, you need to follow an elimination diet that features the beneficial foods discussed in Chapter 4. High-stress foods, such as alcohol, sugar, chocolate, dairy products, red meats, wheat, and convenience foods, should be strictly eliminated from any good antifatigue nutritional program. I had to follow these principles very carefully during my own recovery from chronic fatigue. I spent many weeks eating only foods that clearly did not worsen my fatigue and that actually improved my energy level. This careful attention to what I ate paid real dividends as I finally regained my normal, high level of energy. Over the years I have seen similar elimination diets benefit my patients suffering from fatigue. Particularly in the early stages of recovery, women feel better when they follow these dieting principles—and notably worse if they go back to eating more stressful foods.

I have included in this chapter menus and specific recipes for an antifatigue diet, as well as guidelines on how to make healthy substitutions in your favorite recipes. To make the program easier to use, I have divided the meal plans and recipes into a two-stage program. The first stage is the most restrictive, intended for women with severe fatigue. The meals in this stage are primarily vegetarian based, excluding all or most animal products. However, women whose fatigue is due to anemia may find that they actually feel better if they continue to include small amounts of meat in their diet, especially fish and poultry. This is due to the content of iron and vitamin B_{12} in meat, both necessary nutrients for healthy blood cell formation. Also, while most of my fatigue patients do better in the early stages on a more restricted, vegetarian based diet, I will occasionally encounter women who simply feel better when they include meat in their diets. The meals also primarily contain cooked foods, because many women with chronic fatigue tolerate them better than raw foods. In the second stage, intended for women who are starting to feel better, I have expanded the range of foods by adding some fish dishes, a wider variety of grains, and raw foods such as salads. You can combine these with foods from Stage I. Women with less severe fatigue may want to mix some of the Stage II dishes with the Stage I foods right at the beginning. Remember that *how you feel after eating a meal* is the ultimate test of how you are handling foods. You must become your own feedback system to evaluate whether the foods you have selected are helping to relieve your fatigue and elevate your vitality and well-being.

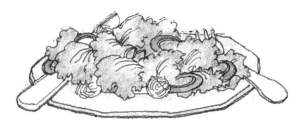

Breakfast Menus

Breakfast is one of the easiest meals to restructure, because it tends to be smaller and simpler and is usually eaten at home. You may want to make the healthful changes in your breakfast first before moving on to lunch and dinner. The breakfast meals in this section are excellent for women who feel extremely tired. I have developed them to give a real boost to your energy levels. The following easy-to-prepare menus provide a good variety of healthful and delicious meals. They can also serve as guidelines to follow when creating your own meal plans. Starred (*) recipes are included in this chapter.

Stage I

Flax shake*   Aloe shake*
Cantaloupe
                         Yam
Banana   Flax oil
Herb tea*   Spring water

Instant flax cereal*
Spring water

Stage II

Millet cereal*   Tofu cereal*
Aloe shake*   Herb tea

Nondairy milk shake*   Brown rice cereal*
                         Fresh carrot juice
Rice cakes
Raw sesame butter
Herb tea

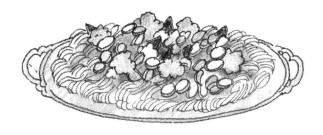

Lunch and Dinner Menus

These menus give you a variety of low-stress, anti-fatigue dishes from which to choose when planning meals. Use these menus while you are healing from your chronic fatigue. Your day-by-day nutritional status can have a significant effect on your vitality and well-being. You can also use these menus as a model for developing your own meal plans. Starred (*) recipes are included in this chapter.

Stage I

Split pea soup*	Potassium broth*
Baked yam*	Kasha*
Steamed kale*	Summer squash and peas*
Vegetable soup*	Lentil soup*
Steamed mustard greens*	Broccoli with lemon*
Baked potato and flax oil*	Millet*
Summer squash soup*	Millet*
Kasha*	Whipped acorn squash*
Steamed carrots*	Steamed green beans
	Cauliflower with flax oil*
Buckwheat pasta	
with flax oil*	Baked yam*
Steamed artichoke*	Brussels sprouts
Vegetable puree #1*	Steamed green peas

Stage II

Hummus*
Raw carrot and
    green pepper sticks
Mixed vegetable salad*

Rice tabouli*
Romaine lettuce salad

Lentils and brown rice
    with flax oil
Steamed artichoke*

Vegetarian taco*
Papaya

Brown rice and pinto beans
Beet salad*
Steamed green peas

Rice cakes
Flax spread*
Apple
Banana

Broiled tuna*
Broccoli with lemon*
Cole slaw*

Poached salmon*
Baked potato*
Steamed kale*

Spinach salad*
Corn muffins*

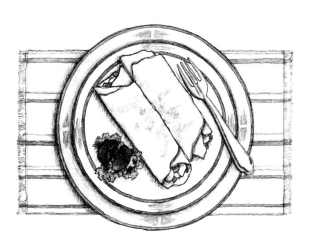

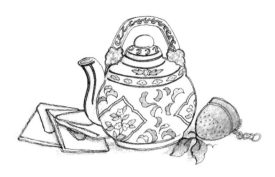

Stage I Recipes: Breakfast

Beverages

These drinks contain specific herbs, fruits, and essential fatty acids that help to combat chronic fatigue. They are low-stress drinks that are easy to absorb and assimilate, and their essential nutrients help energize the body.

Aloe Shake *Serves 2*

1-1/2 cups nondairy milk, plain or vanilla
3 tablespoons flax oil
6 oz. aloe, liquid
3/4 cup frozen berries
1 large banana

Combine all ingredients in a blender. Blend until smooth and serve. Aloe is an herbal liquid that is extremely soothing and easy to digest. It is very well tolerated by women with chronic fatigue.

Energizing Herb Tea *Serves 2*

1 pint water
2 teaspoons grated ginger root
1 teaspoon peppermint leaves

Bring the water to a boil. Place herbs in water and stir. Turn heat to low and steep for 15 minutes. Ginger is a stimulating herb that helps improve your energy level and relieve digestive problems. This drink is an excellent coffee substitute.

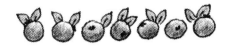

Nondairy Milk Shake *Serves 2*

2 cups nondairy milk,
    vanilla-flavored
3 tablespoons flax oil
1 large banana
3/4 cup frozen berries
    (strawberries, boysen-
    berries, blueberries, or
    raspberries)

Combine all ingredients in a blender. Blend until smooth and serve.

Anti-Stress Herb Tea *Serves 2*

1 pint water
1 teaspoon
    chamomile tea
1 teaspoon
    peppermint leaves

Bring the water to a boil. Place herbs in water and stir. Turn the heat to low and steep for 15 minutes. Chamomile and peppermint are excellent for inducing both emotional and physical relaxation. They are also antispasmodics and help promote better digestive function.

Flax Shake *Serves 2*

6 tablespoons raw
    flax seeds
2 bananas
6 oz. water
6 oz. apple juice or
    nondairy milk

Grind flax seeds to a powder using a coffee or seed grinder. Place powdered flax seeds in a blender. Add remaining ingredients and blend. Whole flax seed is high in essential fatty acids, calcium, magnesium, and potassium.

Cereals

Women commonly have wheat- or dairy-based main courses for breakfast, such as wheat toast, wheat cereal with milk, cottage cheese, and yogurt. As explained in Chapter 4, wheat and dairy products worsen chronic fatigue and tiredness, and should be avoided by women suffering from these symptoms. This section includes recipes for three types of main dishes you can use to replace wheat and dairy products at breakfast. They are based on whole flax seed, soy, and gluten-free grains. (Gluten is the protein found in wheat that can trigger symptoms of fatigue and depression.)

Tofu Cereal　　　　*Serves 2*

4 oz. soft tofu

2 oz. nondairy milk,
　　vanilla-flavored

2 tablespoons flax oil

1 banana

1 apple

5 raw almonds

Combine all ingredients in a food processor. Blend until creamy. Pour into a bowl and serve.

Instant Flax Cereal #1　　*Serves 1*

4 tablespoons
　　raw flax seeds

4 oz. nondairy milk,
　　vanilla-flavored

1/2 banana, sliced

Grind raw flax seeds into a powder using a seed or coffee grinder. Place powder in a cereal bowl and slowly add nondairy milk, stirring the mixture together. The flax mixture will thicken to a texture like cream of rice or oatmeal. Top with sliced banana. Eat the mixture right away because flax seeds are sensitive to light, air, and temperature. Do not cook this cereal; eat it cold. Add more liquid if the cereal thickens too much.

4 tablespoons raw flax
    seeds
4 oz. apple juice
1/8 teaspoon cinnamon

Instant Flax Cereal #2   *Serves 1*

Grind raw flax seeds into a powder using a seed or coffee grinder. Place powder in a cereal bowl and slowly add apple juice and cinnamon, stirring the mixture together. The flax mixture will thicken to a texture like cream of rice or oatmeal. Eat the mixture right away because flax seeds are sensitive to light, air, and temperature. Do not cook this cereal; eat it cold. Add more liquid if the cereal thickens too much.

1 cup millet
2 cups water
1 teaspoon canola oil
4 oz. nondairy milk,
    vanilla-flavored
1/2 banana

Millet Cereal #1   *Serves 2*

Wash millet with cold water. Combine millet, water, and canola oil in a cooking pot. Bring ingredients to a boil. Turn heat to low; cover and cook without stirring for 25–35 minutes, until millet is soft. Resist the temptation to check before 20 minutes, because too much steam will escape. Fluff up the millet and spoon into serving bowls. Add the nondairy milk. Top with sliced banana and serve.

Stage I Recipes:
Lunch and Dinner

Soups

Soups are extremely low-stress foods for women with chronic fatigue. The ingredients are thoroughly cooked and broken down in the soup preparation, so they are easy to absorb and assimilate. The following soups are high in essential nutrients such as potassium and magnesium, which the body needs to combat fatigue. Use these recipes frequently when you have symptoms of severe fatigue.

Vegetable Soup   *Serves 6*

1 onion, chopped
1 stalk celery, chopped
1 turnip, chopped
1/2 leek, chopped
2 carrots, chopped
5 mushrooms, sliced
1 bay leaf
1/2 tablespoon thyme
1/2 tablespoon fennel seeds
1-1/2 quarts water
1/2 teaspoon salt substitute

Place all ingredients in a pot. Bring to a boil, then turn heat to low. Cook for 2 hours. Pour the soup into individual serving dishes.

Lentil Soup   *Serves 4*

1 cup lentils
1/2 onion, chopped
1/2 cup chopped carrots
1 to 1-1/2 quarts water
1 teaspoon brown rice miso

Wash lentils. Put all ingredients in a pot. Bring to a boil, then turn heat to low, cover pot and simmer for 45 minutes or until lentils are soft. Vary the amount of water depending upon the desired thickness of the soup.

1 cup split peas
1/2 onion, chopped
1 small carrot, sliced
1 quart water
1/4 teaspoon sea salt

Split Pea Soup   *Serves 4*

Wash peas. Place peas, onion, and carrot in a pot. Add water. Bring to a boil, then turn heat to low and cover pot. Cook for 45 minutes. Add sea salt and continue to cook until peas are soft. If you prefer a creamy texture, let cool and then puree in a blender.

8 fresh tomatoes
3 cups water
1 cup sliced carrots
1 cup sliced broccoli
1 cup sliced squash
(zucchini or summer
squash)
1/2 cup sliced mushrooms
1/2 cup chopped celery
1 onion, diced
2 garlic cloves, minced
2 tablespoons chopped
fresh parsley
1/4 to 1 teaspoon fresh or
dried basil (to taste)

Potassium Broth   *Serves 8 to 10*

Liquefy tomatoes in a blender. Combine all ingredients in soup pot and bring to a boil. Turn heat to low and simmer for 2 hours. Strain and serve.

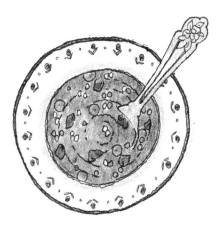

Summer Squash Soup *Serves 6*

4 yellow summer squash, chopped
1 onion, chopped
1 quart water
1/4 to 1/2 teaspoon sea salt (miso or tamari may be substituted)

Place chopped squash and onion in a pot. Add water and bring to a boil. Turn heat to low and cover pot; cook for 15 minutes. Add sea salt and continue cooking for another 15 minutes, until vegetables are soft. Cool and then puree in blender. Garnish with sliced scallions or minced parsley.

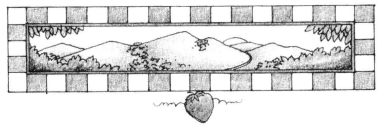

Grains and Starches

Because starches are so easily digested, women with chronic fatigue may eat them even in the early stages of treatment. As your energy begins to pick up and your fatigue becomes less severe, you may add nongluten-containing grains.

Baked Potato *Serves 4*

4 russet or Idaho potatoes
1 tablespoon vegetable oil
2 tablespoons flax oil for each potato

Preheat oven to 400°F. Wash potatoes, rub with vegetable oil, and bake for 45–60 minutes, or until soft when pierced with a fork. Mash insides and mix with flax oil, if desired. Flax oil has a delicious buttery flavor and I highly recommend that you try it!

Baked Yams
Serves 4

4 yams
2 tablespoons flax oil
for each yam

Preheat oven to 400°F. Wash yams and bake for 45–60 minutes, or until soft when pierced with a fork. Top with flax oil, if desired.

Kasha
Serves 4

1 cup kasha (buckwheat groats)
3-1/4 cups water
pinch salt

Bring ingredients to a boil, lower heat, and simmer for 25 minutes or until soft. The grains should be fluffy, like rice. For breakfast, blend in blender with water until creamy. Add almond milk, sesame milk, or sunflower milk, and cinnamon, apple butter, ginger, raisins, or berries.

Millet
Serves 2

1 cup millet
2 cups cold water
1/2 teaspoon sea salt

Wash millet with cold water. Combine all ingredients in a cooking pot. Bring to a rapid boil. Turn heat to low, cover, and cook without stirring until millet is soft (about 25–35 minutes). Resist the temptation to check before 20 minutes, because too much steam will escape.

Vegetables

Summer Squash and Peas

Serves 4

2 to 3 small summer
squash, diced
1 cup peas

Steam peas for 10 minutes. Add squash and steam vegetables together for 15 minutes, or until tender. Drain and serve.

Vegetable Puree #1 *Serves 4*

3 to 4 carrots, chopped
1/8 head cabbage, chopped
1 cup peas

Steam carrots for 15 minutes, add rest of vegetables, and steam another 15 minutes, until soft. Place in blender and puree. Slowly add water until smooth and creamy.

Vegetable Puree #2 *Serves 4*

4 summer squash, chopped
1 medium beet, chopped

Steam beet for 15 minutes. Add squash to the pot and steam vegetables together for 15 minutes, or until soft. Puree in blender.

Cauliflower with Flax Oil

Serves 4

1 medium head cauliflower
4 tablespoons flax oil
1 teaspoon salt substitute

Break cauliflower into small flowerets. Steam 10 minutes or until tender. Toss with flax oil and salt substitute and serve.

Broccoli with Lemon *Serves 4*

1 pound broccoli
juice of 1/2 lemon
4 tablespoons flax oil

Cut the broccoli into small flowerets. Steam 12 minutes or until tender. Squeeze lemon juice over broccoli and add flax oil. Mix and serve.

Steamed Kale *Serves 4*

1 bunch kale
juice of 1 lemon
1 teaspoon olive oil
pinch sea salt

Strip kale leaves from the stems and discard the stems. Wash leaves and place in a steamer. Steam 12 minutes or until tender. Dress with lemon juice, olive oil, and sea salt.

Steamed Carrots *Serves 4*

12 small carrots, sliced
1 teaspoon maple syrup

Steam carrots until soft. Drizzle with maple syrup if desired.

Steamed Zucchini *Serves 4*

2 medium zucchini, diced
2 teaspoons scallions

Steam zucchini for 4–6 minutes. Sprinkle with chopped scallions and serve.

Whipped Acorn Squash *Serves 4*

2 acorn squash
2–3 oz. apple juice
pinch ground cinnamon

Peel and cut acorn squash into large pieces. Steam until tender. Place in food processor, add apple juice and cinnamon, and puree. You may also want to add water in small amounts until smooth and creamy.

4 artichokes

Steamed Artichokes   *Serves 4*

Trim the artichokes. Place them in a steamer with sufficient water to steam for 45 minutes. Remove from steamer and serve hot or cold. Use with flax oil as a dip, if desired.

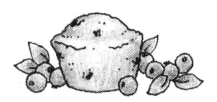

Stage II Recipes: Breakfast

Cereals and Muffins

The following breakfast foods are suitable for women who are in later recovery from chronic fatigue or who have less severe symptoms. These recipes use highly nutritious ingredients that are somewhat more difficult to break down and digest than the Stage I foods.

1 cup millet
2 cups water
1 teaspoon canola oil
4 oz. nondairy milk, vanilla-flavored
1 teaspoon raw sunflower seeds
1 teaspoon raw sesame seeds

Millet Cereal #2   *Serves 2*

Wash millet with cold water. Combine millet, 2 cups water, and canola oil in a pot. Bring to a boil. Turn heat to low, cover, and cook without stirring about 25–35 minutes, until millet is soft. Don't check before 20 minutes, because too much stream will escape. Fluff up millet and spoon into serving bowls. Add remaining ingredients. Mix and serve.

Brown Rice Cereal *Serves 2*

1 cup brown rice
2 cups water
pinch sea salt
1 tablespoon raisins
20 raw almonds
2 oz. nondairy milk,
    vanilla-flavored,
    or apple juice

Wash rice in cold water. Combine rice, 2 cups water, and salt in a pot. Bring to a boil. Stir and turn heat to low. Cover pot and cook without stirring about 25–35 minutes. Don't open pot and check before 20 minutes, because too much steam will escape. Add remaining ingredients. Mix and serve.

Corn Muffins *Serves 8 to 10*

2 tablespoons canola oil
3 tablespoons honey
2 eggs, beaten
2 cups nondairy milk,
    vanilla-flavored
2 cups cornmeal
1/2 cup rice flour
1/2 teaspoon salt
1 teaspoon baking powder
1/2 teaspoon baking soda

Combine oil, honey, eggs, and nondairy milk in a bowl; mix well and set aside. Mix together corn-meal, rice flour, salt, baking powder, and baking soda. Combine wet and dry ingredients and mix until batter is smooth. Spoon into well-oiled muffin tins and bake about 20 minutes at 425°F. Delicious with fresh flax oil (a fine butter replacement) or blackberry preserves and raw almond butter.

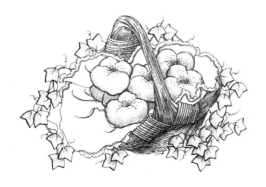

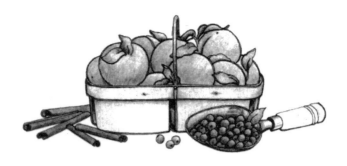

Stage II Recipes:
Lunch and Dinner

Spreads and Sauces

These spreads contain highly nutritious ingredients. Eat with rice bread, crackers, corn bread, or even spread on a banana for a delicious treat.

Flax Spread *Serves 2*

4 tablespoons raw flax seeds
juice of 1/2 lemon
1/2 teaspoon Bragg's
   Liquid Amino Acids
2 tablespoons water

Grind flax seeds to a powder using a coffee or seed grinder. Add remaining ingredients and mix into a paste. Use as a spread with rice cakes or crackers. Use additional water if spread becomes too thick.

Fresh Applesauce *Serves 2*

1/2 cup fresh apple juice
2-1/2 apples
1/2 teaspoon cinnamon

Peel apples and cut into quarters. Combine all ingredients in a food processor. Blend until smooth.

Salads

These are excellent salads for women with fatigue who can handle raw foods. They are high in vitamins and minerals and contain no eggs or dairy products. Try them for a delicious addition to your meals.

Mixed Vegetable Salad

Serves 4 to 6

1 head green or
   red leaf lettuce
1/2 cup chopped broccoli,
   steamed
1/2 cup chopped green beans,
   steamed
1 small raw carrot, sliced
1 large tomato, sliced
1/4 small red onion, chopped
1/4 cup raw mixed bean sprouts

Combine all ingredients in a large salad bowl. Serve with an oil-and-vinegar dressing (be sure to avoid cheese or cream dressings).

Spinach Salad   *Serves 4*

1 bunch spinach, chopped
1/2 small red onion, chopped
1/3 cup red pepper, diced
1/2 cup mung bean sprouts
2 oz. firm tofu, diced
1/4 cup raw sunflower seeds

Combine all ingredients in a large salad bowl. Serve with your favorite nondairy dressing.

Beet Salad   *Serves 4*

3 medium-sized beets,
   diced and steamed
1 red onion, chopped
1/2 bunch parsley, chopped
1/2 red pepper, diced
1/4 cup sunflower seeds

Combine all ingredients in a large salad bowl. Serve with an oil-and-vinegar dressing (avoid cheese or cream dressings). This salad is great in summer.

Potato Salad *Serves 6*

8 medium-sized red potatoes
1 cup chopped celery
1/2 cup finely chopped parsley
1/2 cup chopped green pepper
1/2 cup chopped sweet, raw onions

Steam potatoes for approximately 45 minutes. Cool and cube. Combine celery, parsley, pepper, and onions with potatoes; mix thoroughly. Add a small amount of your favorite dressing. Both vinaigrette and low-calorie mayonnaise are delicious on potato salad.

Cole Slaw *Serves 4*

1/2 teaspoon celery seeds
1/2 teaspoon poppy seeds
1/2 teaspoon dill
2 cups finely shredded red cabbage
1-1/2 cups finely shredded green cabbage

Crush or grind the seeds; add, with dill, to shredded cabbage. Serve with your favorite dressing (oil-and-vinegar or honey dressing preferred). The seeds and dill are high in calcium, magnesium, and iron.

Grains and Starches

Brown Rice *Serves 4*

1 cup brown rice
2 cups cold water
1/2 teaspoon sea salt

Wash rice with cold water. Combine rice, 2 cups cold water, and salt in a cooking pot. Bring to a rapid boil. Turn heat to low, cover, and cook without stirring until rice is soft (about 25–35 minutes). Resist the temptation to check before 20 minutes, because too much steam will escape.

Adzuki Beans *Serves 4*

1 cup adzuki beans
4 cups water
1/4 teaspoon sea salt

Wash beans. Place in a pot with the water and salt. Bring to a boil, cover, and simmer for 2 hours or until beans are tender.

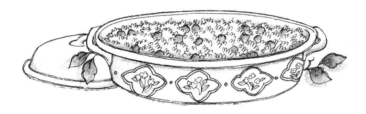

Main Dishes

These dishes use grains, legumes, or fish as primary ingredients. The recipes are easy to make and delicious. They provide high-nutrient main dishes to women experiencing mild to moderate fatigue.

Rice Tabouli *Serves 6*

2 cups cooked brown rice
1 cup chopped parsley
1/2 cup chopped fresh mint
1/2 red onion, diced
1 medium tomato, diced
juice of 1 lemon
2 tablespoons olive oil
1 teaspoon cumin
1 teaspoon oregano
1/4 teaspoon salt

Place rice in a bowl. Mix in parsley, mint, red onion, and tomato. Combine well. Add lemon juice and olive oil and mix again. Add cumin, oregano, and salt to the salad; mix well. This is the ultimate delicious and healthy tabouli recipe. It is great with hummus (following).

3/4 cup raw unhulled
sesame seeds
1 cup water or cooking
liquid from beans
1-3/4 cup garbanzo beans,
cooked
juice of 1 lemon
2 tablespoons olive oil
1 clove raw garlic
1/4 teaspoon salt

Hummus
Serves 4

Grind sesame seeds into a powder using a seed or coffee grinder. (Raw sesame butter, which is available from most health food stores, may be substituted for the ground sesame seeds.) Combine ground sesame seeds with water, garbanzo beans, lemon juice, olive oil, garlic, and salt in a food processor. Blend to the consistency of a smooth dip. Serve as a dip with pita bread, rye bread, and fresh vegetables. This is great served with rice tabouli (see preceding recipe).

Tofu and Almond Stir-Fry
Serves 4

3/4 cup firm tofu, cubed
1 cup chopped raw almonds
1/4 yellow onion, chopped
1/2 red pepper, chopped
1/4 cup water
1 teaspoon sesame or
safflower oil
3 cups cooked brown rice
1 teaspoon wheat-free
soy sauce (tamari)

Combine tofu, almonds, onion, and red pepper in a large frying pan with water and oil. Cook over low heat for 5 minutes. (Add extra water to pan if needed.) Add cooked rice and mix. Heat for 5 minutes or until warm. Transfer to serving dish and toss with wheat-free soy sauce.

4 corn tortillas
3/4 pound pinto beans,
    cooked and pureed
1/2 avocado, thinly sliced
1/4 sweet red pepper, diced
1 tomato, diced
1/4 red onion,
    finely chopped
1/2 head red or romaine
    lettuce, chopped
6 tablespoons salsa

Vegetarian Tacos   *Serves 4*

Warm tortillas and beans in separate pans. Place tortillas on individual serving dishes and spread with beans. Garnish with avocado, pepper, tomato, and onion; then cover each taco with lettuce and 1-1/2 tablespoons of salsa.

1 cup water
juice of 1 lemon
4 fillets of salmon,
    3 oz. each

Poached Salmon   *Serves 4*

Combine water and lemon juice in skillet and heat. Place salmon in hot liquid. Cover and poach for 6 to 8 minutes or until salmon flakes easily with a fork. Remove fish and keep it warm until you are ready to serve.

4 fillets of tuna, 4 oz. each
1 tablespoon canola oil
2 tablespoons lemon juice

Broiled Tuna   *Serves 4*

Baste tuna fillets with oil and sprinkle with lemon juice. Place tuna in a broiler pan. Broil for 5–6 minutes, or until done to your satisfaction.

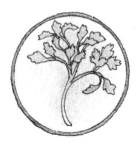

Substitute Healthy Ingredients in Recipes

Learning how to make substitutions for high-stress ingredients in familiar recipes allows you to make your favorite foods without compromising your energy level and vitality. Many recipes contain ingredients that women with chronic fatigue must avoid—dairy products, alcohol, sugar, chocolate, wheat flour. By eliminating the high-stress foods and replacing them with healthier ingredients, you can continue to make many recipes that appeal to you. I have recommended this approach for years to my patients, who are pleased to find that they can still have their favorite dishes, but in much healthier versions.

Some women choose to totally eliminate high-stress ingredients from a recipe. For example, you can make a pasta with tomato sauce, but eliminate the Parmesan cheese topping and use nonwheat pasta. Greek salad can be made without the feta cheese. Some of my patients even make pizza without cheese, layering tomato sauce and lots of vegetables on the crust. In many cases, the high-stress ingredients are not necessary to make foods taste good; always remember, they can worsen your fatigue symptoms.

If you want to retain a particular high-stress ingredient, you can usually substantially reduce the amount of that ingredient you use, while still retaining the flavor and taste. Most of us have palates jaded by too much fat, salt, sugar, and other flavorings. In many dishes, we taste only the additives; we never really enjoy the delicious flavors of the foods themselves. Now that I regularly substitute low-stress ingredients in my cooking, I find that I enjoy the subtle taste of the dishes much more. Also, I find that my health and vitality continue to improve with the deletion of high-stress ingredients from my food. The following information tells you how to substitute healthy ingredients in your own recipes. The substitutions are simple to make and should benefit your health greatly.

How to Substitute for Caffeinated Foods and Beverages

Drink substitutes for coffee and black tea. The best substitutes are the grain-based coffee beverages, such as Pero, Postum, and Caffix. Some women may find the abrupt discontinuance of coffee too difficult because of withdrawal symptoms, such as headaches. If this concerns you, decrease your total coffee intake gradually to only one or one-half cup per day. Use coffee substitutes for your other cups. This will help prevent withdrawal symptoms.

Use decaffeinated coffee or tea as a transition beverage. If you cannot give up coffee, start by substituting water-processed decaffeinated coffee for the real thing. Then try to wean yourself from coffee altogether, or go to a coffee substitute.

Use herbal teas for energy and vitality. Many women with chronic fatigue mistakenly drink coffee as a pick-me-up to be able to function during the day. Use ginger instead. It is a great herbal stimulant that won't wreck your health. To make ginger tea, grate a few teaspoons of fresh ginger root into a pot of hot water; boil and steep. Serve with honey.

Substitute carob for chocolate. Unsweetened carob tastes like chocolate but is far more nutritious. A member of the legume family, carob is high in calcium. You can purchase it in chunk form as a substitute for chocolate candy or as a powder for use in baking or drinks. Be careful, however, not to overindulge; carob, like chocolate, is high in calories and fat. Consider it a treat and an excellent cooking aid for use in small amounts only.

How to Substitute for Sugar

Substitute concentrated sweeteners. Americans tend to be addicted to sugar. Most of us grew up on highly sugared soft drinks, candy, and rich pastries—no wonder the incidence of diabetes is soaring among our population. I have found that as women decrease their sugar intake, most begin to really enjoy the subtle flavors of the foods they eat. Concentrated sweeteners such as honey and maple syrup have a sweeter taste per quantity used than table sugar. Using these substitutes will allow you to decrease the actual amount of sugar you use in a recipe. If you use a concentrated sweetener in place of sugar in an ordinary recipe, reduce the liquid content in the recipe by one-fourth cup. If no liquid is used in the recipe, add 3 to 5 tablespoons of flour for each three-fourths cup of concentrated sweetener.

Substitute fruit for sugar in pastries. In making muffins and cookies, you may want to try deleting sugar altogether and adding extra fruits and nuts.

How to Substitute for Alcohol

Use low-alcohol or nonalcoholic products for cooking. Substitute low-alcohol or nonalcoholic wine or beer when cooking or preparing sauces and marinades. You will retain much of the flavor that alcohol imparts, and you'll decrease the stress factor substantially.

How to Substitute for Dairy Products

Eliminate or decrease the amount of cow's milk cheese you use in food preparation and cooking. If you must use cow's milk cheese in cooking, decrease the amount in the recipe by three-fourths so that it becomes a flavoring or garnish rather than a major source of fat and protein. For example, use one teaspoon of Parmesan cheese on top of a casserole instead of one-half cup.

Use soy cheese in food preparation and cooking. Soy cheese is an excellent substitute for cow's milk cheese. It is lower in fat and salt, and the fat it does contain isn't saturated. Women with severe fatigue may have difficulty digesting it, so I recommend its use with women who are recovering from their chronic fatigue symptoms. Health food stores offer many brands that come in many different flavors, such as mozzarella, cheddar, American, and jack. The quality of these products keeps improving all the time. You can use soy cheese as a perfect cheese substitute in sandwiches, salads, pizzas, lasagnas, and casseroles. In some recipes you can replace cheese with soft tofu. I have done this often with lasagna, layering the lasagna noodles with tofu and topping with melted soy cheese for a delicious dish. The tofu, which is bland, takes on the taste of the tomato sauce.

Replace milk in recipes. For cow's milk, substitute potato milk, soy milk, nut milk, or grain milk. One of my personal favorites is a nondairy milk that is made from an all-vegetable potato base. It is easily digestible and particularly good for women with chronic fatigue. It is creamy and sweet and tastes very similar to the best cow's milk, with none of the unhealthy characteristics of dairy products. Even my 10-year-old daughter likes it. The potato-based milk is high in calcium and can be bought dry so that you can store it. It mixes easily in water and can be used exactly as you use cow's milk for beverages, cooking, and baking. Potato milk is available through *The LIFECYCLES Center.* Soy milk and nut milk are available at most health food stores. Soy milk is particularly good and comes in many flavors. Many nondairy milks are good sources of calcium and can be used for drinking, eating, or baking.

Substitute flax oil for butter. Flax oil is the best substitute for butter that I've found. It is a rich, golden oil that looks and tastes quite a bit like butter. It is delicious on anything you'd normally top with butter—toast, rice, popcorn, steamed vegetables, or potatoes. Flax oil is extremely high in essential fatty acids—the type of fat that is very healthy for a woman's body. Essential fatty acids improve vitality, enhance circulation, and help promote normal hormonal function. Flax oil is quite perishable, however, because it is sensitive to heat and light. You can't cook with it—cook the food first and add the flax oil before serving. Also, keep it refrigerated. Flax oil has so many health benefits that I highly recommend its use. You can find it in health food stores or order it through *The LIFECYCLES Center* if there is no health food store near you.

How to Substitute for Red Meat and Poultry

Substitute beans, tofu, or seeds in recipes. You can often modify recipes calling for hamburger or ground turkey by substituting tofu. For example, crumble up the tofu to simulate the texture of hamburger and add to recipes for enchiladas, tacos, chili, and ground beef casseroles. The tofu takes on the flavor of the sauce used in the dish and is indistinguishable from meat. I do this often when cooking at home.

When making salads that call for meat, such as chef's salad or Cobb salad, substitute kidney beans and garbanzo beans, along with sunflower seeds. These will provide the needed protein, yet be more easily digestible. You can also sprinkle sunflower seeds on top of casseroles for extra protein and essential fatty acids. When making stir-fries, substitute tofu, almonds, or sprouts for beef or chicken. Vegetable protein-based stir-fries taste delicious!

How to Substitute for Wheat Flour

Use whole grain, nonwheat flour. Substitute whole grain, nonwheat flours, such as rice or barley flour. Whole grain flours are much higher in essential nutrients, such as the vitamin B complex and many minerals. They are also higher in fiber content. Rice flour makes excellent cookies, cakes, and other pastries. Barley flour is best used for pie crusts.

How to Substitute for Salt

Substitute potassium-based products for table salt (sodium chloride). Potassium-based products, such as Morton's Salt Substitute, are much healthier and will not aggravate heart disease or hypertension.

Use powdered seaweeds such as kelp or nori to season vegetables, grains, and salads. They are high in essential iodine and trace elements.

Use herbs instead of salt for flavoring. Their flavors are much more subtle and will help even the most jaded palate appreciate the taste of fresh fruits, vegetables, and meats.

Use liquid flavoring agents with advertised low-sodium content. Low-salt soy sauce and Bragg's Amino Acids, a liquid soybean-based flavoring agent, are delicious when used as salt substitutes in cooking. Add them to soups, casseroles, stir-fries, and other dishes at the end of the cooking process. You will find that you need only a small amount for intense flavoring.

Substitutes for Common High-Stress Ingredients

3/4 cup sugar	1/2 cup honey 1/4 cup molasses 1/2 cup maple syrup 1/2 oz. barley malt 1 cup apple butter 2 cups apple juice
1 cup milk	1 cup soy, potato, nut, or grain milk
1 tablespoon butter	1 tablespoon flax oil (must be used raw and unheated)
1/2 teaspoon salt	1 tablespoon miso 1/2 teaspoon potassium chloride salt substitute 1/2 teaspoon Mrs. Dash, Spike 1/2 teaspoon herbs (basil, tarragon, oregano, etc.)
1-1/2 cups cocoa	1 cup powdered carob
1 square chocolate	3/4 tablespoon powdered carob
1 tablespoon coffee	1 tablespoon decaffeinated coffee 1 tablespoon Pero, Postum, Caffix, or other grain-based coffee substitute
4 oz. wine	4 oz. light wine
8 oz. beer	8 oz. near beer
1 cup wheat flour	1 cup barley flour (pie crust) 1 cup rice flour (cookies, cakes, breads)
1 cup meat	1 cup beans, tofu 1/4 cup seeds

6

Vitamins, Minerals, & Herbs

*N*utritional supplements can play an important role in your chronic fatigue recovery program. They help stimulate your immune system, glands, and digestive tract, and they can help stabilize and relax your mood. They also promote good circulation of blood and oxygen to the entire body, a necessity for high energy and vitality. When adequate nutritional support is lacking, I have found it very difficult to entirely relieve fatigue. In fact, poor or inadequate nutrition may play a major role in causing fatigue. Thus, the use of essential nutrients is an important facet of a good chronic fatigue treatment program. Numerous research studies done at university centers and hospitals support the importance of nutrition in relieving fatigue; a bibliography is included at the end of this chapter for those wanting more technical information.

Most women have difficulty getting their nutrient intake up to the levels needed for optimal healing using diet alone. The use of supplements can help make up this deficiency so you can heal as rapidly and completely as possible. I do want to emphasize the importance of a good diet along with the use of supplements. Supplements should never be used as an excuse to continue poor dietary habits. I have found that my patients heal most effectively when they combine a nutrient-rich diet with the right mix of supplements.

This chapter is divided into four sections. The first discusses the role of vitamins and minerals; the second section explains the beneficial effects of fatty acids. The third section tells which herbs help relieve chronic fatigue. I end the chapter with specific recommendations on how to make and use your own supplements, along with a series of charts that list major food sources for each essential nutrient.

Vitamins and Minerals for Chronic Fatigue

Many vitamins and minerals are useful in the treatment and prevention of fatigue. While a high-nutrient diet plays an important role in combating fatigue, you may get the best therapeutic results by adding supplements to boost the level of these nutrients. However, I must caution you to use supplements very carefully. This chapter includes formulas with specific dosage recommendations for supplements, but I suggest that you start slowly. You may want to begin with as little as one-fourth of the listed dose, to see how you tolerate the supplements. You can then increase your dose gradually until you find the level that works best for you. Very rarely, women experience nausea or diarrhea when beginning a supplement program. If this happens, your body is having difficulty tolerating a particular supplement. In this case, stop all supplements. After a week you may want to begin your supplement intake again. Start with one supplement at a time until you discover which one gives you trouble. You should probably eliminate that supplement from your program. Before taking any supplements, consult your physician or a nutritionist with specific questions about their use or possible side effects.

Vitamin A. This nutrient helps protect the body against invasion by pathogens such as viruses (which might trigger chronic fatigue syndrome) and by bacteria, fungi, and allergies. It does this in several ways. Vitamin A supports the production and maintenance of healthy skin, as well as the mucous membranes that line the mouth, lungs, digestive tract, bladder, and cervix. When these tissues are healthy, invaders have difficulty penetrating the membranes, the body's first line of defense. Vitamin A also enhances the immune system by increasing T-cell activity (these are important cells that help to fight infectious disease). Vitamin A also contributes to the health of the thymus, a gland located in the chest that plays an important role in maintaining healthy immune function.

Because Vitamin A is needed for normal production of red blood cells, it helps prevent fatigue caused by anemia. It also helps control the tiredness caused by anemia that occurs with heavy menstrual bleeding.

Vitamin A should be used carefully. It is a fat-soluble vitamin that is stored in the body. You should not take more than 20,000 I.U. (international units) per day without being monitored by a physician. An overdose of vitamin A can cause headaches and stress the liver.

Beta carotene, called provitamin A, is a precursor of vitamin A found in fruits and vegetables. Beta carotene is water-soluble and, unlike vitamin A, does not accumulate in the body. As a result, it can be used safely in high doses. Certain foods, such as sweet potatoes and carrots, contain large amounts of beta carotene. A single sweet potato or a cup of fresh carrot juice contains 25,000 I.U. of beta carotene.

Provitamin A also enhances immune function. It stimulates immune cells called macrophages and helps trigger increased immune activity against certain bacteria as well as candida. Beta carotene is also a powerful antioxidant that helps to protect the body from damage by free radicals. Free radicals are chemicals that occur as by-products of oxygen use in the body, exposure to ultraviolet light, and other natural processes; they can damage the cell membranes as well as other parts of the cell. Antioxidants like beta carotene neutralize free radicals.

Vitamin B Complex. This complex consists of 11 vitamin B factors. The whole complex works together to perform important metabolic functions, including glucose metabolism, stabilization of brain chemistry, and inactivation of estrogen. These processes regulate the body's level of energy and vitality. Because B vitamins are water-soluble and are not stored in the body, they are easily lost when a woman is under stress or is eating unhealthy food, including coffee, cola drinks, and other caffeine-containing beverages. Fatigue and depression can result from the depletion of B vitamins.

Many women with anemia are deficient in three B-complex vitamins—folic acid, pyridoxine (vitamin B_6), and vitamin B_{12}. All three are needed for normal growth and maturation of red blood cells. Their deficiency leads to anemia and fatigue. Supplemental vitamin B_{12} is necessary for women on a vegetarian diet. It is usually given by injection.

Vitamin B_6 is extremely important in relieving and preventing fatigue. In women who are prone to fatigue caused by bacteria, viruses, candida, or allergies, B_6 supports a healthy immune response. B_6 is needed for both the production of antibodies by white blood cells and the production of T-cell lymphocytes by the thymus. This vitamin also appears to help enhance the activity of the T-cells, making them more effective in destroying infectious agents.

Vitamin B_6 helps reduce PMS-related mood swings, fatigue, food cravings, and fluid retention through its effect on glucose metabolism and its participation in prostaglandin synthesis. Prostaglandins—hormones that regulate many important physiological functions—are formed in the body from certain essential vegetable and fish oils. The essential fats can only be converted to prostaglandins in the presence of B_6 and other essential nutrients. Prostaglandin deficiency adversely affects brain chemistry and mood and can worsen fatigue.

Women using birth control pills and menopausal women on hormonal replacement therapy can be prone to fatigue because the use of hormones causes vitamin B_6 deficiency. Finally, B_6 deficiency has been found in fatigued women who suffer from depression. Vitamin B_6 can be taken safely by most women in doses up to 250 milligrams. Doses above this level should be avoided because B_6 can cause toxic symptoms in the nervous system in susceptible women. The B-complex vitamins are usually found together in beans and whole grains. These foods should be part of the diet of women with chronic fatigue, who would also probably benefit from the use of supplemental vitamin B.

Vitamin C. This an extremely important nutrient for fatigue. In one research study done on 411 dentists and their spouses, scientists found a clear relationship between the presence of fatigue and lack of vitamin C. By supporting the immune function, vitamin C helps prevent fatigue caused by infections. It stimulates the production of interferon, a chemical found to prevent the spread of viruses in the body. Necessary for healthy white blood cells and their antibody production, vitamin C also helps the body fight bacterial and fungal infections. Women with low vitamin-C intake tend to have elevated levels of histamine, a chemical that triggers allergy symptoms. Vitamin C is an important antistress vitamin, needed for the production of sufficient adrenal gland hormones. Healthy adrenal function helps prevent fatigue and exhaustion in women who are under physical or emotional stress.

In women with iron deficiency anemia, vitamin C increases the absorption of iron from the digestive tract. Vitamin C has also been tested, along with bioflavonoids, as a treatment for anemia caused by heavy menstrual bleeding—a common cause of fatigue in teenagers and premenopausal women in their forties. Vitamin C reduces bleeding by helping to strengthen capillaries and prevent capillary fragility. One clinical study of vitamin C showed a reduction in bleeding in 87 percent of women taking supplemental amounts of this essential nutrient.

The best sources of vitamin C in nature are fruits and vegetables. It is a water-soluble vitamin, so it is not stored in the body. Thus, women with chronic fatigue should replenish their vitamin C supply daily through a healthy diet and the use of supplements.

Bioflavonoids. These nutrients are found abundantly in flowers and in fruits, particularly oranges, grapefruits, cherries, huckleberries, blackberries, and grape skins. Besides giving pigmentation to plants, they have a number of beneficial physiological effects that can help decrease fatigue symptoms. Bioflavonoids are powerful antioxidants that help protect cells against damage by free radicals.

They help protect us from fatigue caused by allergic reactions, because their anti-inflammatory properties help prevent the production and release of compounds such as histamine and leukotrienes that promote inflammation. Bioflavonoids such as quercetin have powerful antiviral properties that protect us from infections. Quercetin also inhibits the release of allergic compounds from mast cells—the cells in the digestive and respiratory tract that release histamine.

Bioflavonoids are among the most important nutrients for mid-life women suffering from menopausal symptoms. Bioflavonoids produce chemical activity similar to estrogen and can be used as an estrogen substitute. Clinical studies have shown that bioflavonoids can help control hot flashes and the psychological symptoms of menopause, including fatigue, irritability, and mood swings. Interestingly, bioflavonoids contain a very low potency of estrogen, much lower than that used in hormonal replacement therapy. As a result, no harmful side effects have been noted with bioflavonoid therapy.

Because of their ability to strengthen capillary walls, bioflavonoids have also shown dramatic results in reducing the anemia caused by heavy menstrual bleeding. They have been used in women with bleeding caused by hormonal imbalance and have even been tested in women who have lost multiple pregnancies because of bleeding. They were used in conjunction with vitamin C in these studies. Bioflavonoids are often found with vitamin C in fruits and vegetables.

Vitamin E. This vitamin can enhance immune antibody response at high levels and has a significant immune stimulation effect. Vitamin E has antihistamine properties and should be used by women who suffer from allergies. One group of volunteers who were injected with histamine showed far less allergic swelling around the injection site when they were pretreated with vitamin E.

Like vitamin C and beta carotene, vitamin E is an important antioxidant. It protects the cells from the destructive effects of environmental pollutants that can react with the cell membrane. Because it has been found to increase red blood cell survival, it is an important nutrient for the prevention of anemia.

Vitamin E can act as an estrogen substitute. Like bioflavonoids, it has been studied as a treatment for hot flashes and for the psychological symptoms of menopause, including depression and fatigue. It can even relieve vaginal dryness in those women who either can't take or can't tolerate estrogen. According to one study, vitamin E helped skew the progesterone/estrogen ratio in the body toward progesterone. This could be very helpful for women who have heavy menstrual bleeding caused by excess estrogen. Vitamin E is also needed for healthy thyroid function.

Vitamin E occurs in abundance in wheat germ, nuts, seeds, and some fruits and vegetables.

Iron. An essential component of red blood cells, iron combines with protein and copper to make hemoglobin, the pigment of the red blood cells. Studies have shown that women with iron deficiency have decreased physical stamina and endurance. Iron deficiency, the main cause of anemia, is common during all phases of a woman's life, because of both poor nutritional habits and regular blood loss through menstruation. Iron deficiency frequently causes fatigue and low energy states.

Women who suffer from heavy menstrual bleeding are more likely to be iron deficient than woman with normal menstrual flow. In fact, some medical studies have found that inadequate iron intake may be a cause of excessive bleeding as well as an effect of the problem. Women who suffer from heavy menstrual bleeding should have their red blood count checked to see if supplemental iron and a high-iron diet are necessary.

Good sources of iron include liver, blackstrap molasses, beans and peas, seeds and nuts, and certain fruits and vegetables. The body absorbs and assimilates the *heme iron* from meat sources, such as liver, much better than the *non-heme iron* from vegetarian sources. To absorb non-heme iron properly, you must take it with at least 75 milligrams of vitamin C.

Zinc. Zinc plays an important role in combating fatigue. Supplementation with zinc improves muscle strength and endurance. It reduces fatigue by enhancing immune function, acting as an immune stimulant and triggering the reproduction of lymphocytes when incubated with these cells in a test tube. Zinc is a constituent of many enzymes involved in both metabolism and digestion. It is needed for the proper growth and development of female reproductive organs and for the normal functioning of the male prostate gland. Good food sources of zinc include wheat germ, pumpkin seeds, whole-grain wheat bran, and high-protein foods.

Magnesium. Adequate levels of this essential mineral are very important for the maintenance of energy and vitality. Magnesium is required for the production of ATP, the end product of the conversion of food to usable energy by the body's cells. ATP is the universal energy currency that the body uses to run hundreds of thousands of chemical reactions. This energy can be efficiently extracted from food only in the presence of magnesium, oxygen, and other nutrients. Medical research studies in the treatment of chronic fatigue use a special form of magnesium called magnesium aspartate, formed by combining magnesium with aspartic acid. Aspartic acid also plays an important role in the production of energy in the body and helps transport magnesium and potassium into the cells. Magnesium aspartate, along with potassium aspartate, has been tested in a number of clinical studies and has been shown to dramatically improve energy levels after five to six weeks of constant use. Many volunteers began to feel better even within ten days. This beneficial effect was seen in 90 percent of the people tested, a very high success rate.

Magnesium is an important nutrient for women with chronic

candida infections. A magnesium deficiency can develop from the diarrhea, vomiting, and other digestive problems associated with intestinal candida infections. Magnesium deficiency can worsen fatigue, weakness, confusion, and muscle tremor in women with candida infections. Women with these symptoms must replace the magnesium through appropriate supplementation. Magnesium deficiency has also been seen in women suffering from PMS; medical studies have found a reduction in red blood cell magnesium during the second half of the menstrual cycle in affected women. Magnesium, like vitamin B_6, is needed for the production of the beneficial prostaglandin hormones as well as for glucose metabolism. Magnesium supplements can also benefit women with severe emotional stress, anxiety, and insomnia. When taken before bedtime, magnesium helps to calm the mood and induce restful sleep. Good food sources of magnesium include green leafy vegetables, beans and peas, raw nuts and seeds, tofu, avocado, raisins, dried figs, millet and other grains.

Potassium. Like magnesium, potassium has a powerful enhancing effect on energy and vitality. Potassium deficiency has been associated with fatigue and muscular weakness. One study showed that older people who were deficient in potassium had weaker grip strength. Potassium aspartate has been used with magnesium aspartate in a number of studies on chronic fatigue; this combination significantly restored energy levels.

Potassium has many important roles in the body. It regulates the transfer of nutrients into the cells and works with sodium to maintain the body's water balance. Its role in water balance is important in preventing PMS bloating symptoms. Potassium aids proper muscle contraction and transmission of electrochemical impulses. It helps maintain nervous system function and a healthy heart rate. Potassium is found in abundance in fruits, vegetables, beans and peas, seeds and nuts, starches, and whole grains.

Calcium. This mineral helps combat stress, nervous tension, and anxiety. An upset emotional state can dramatically worsen fatigue in susceptible women. A calcium deficiency worsens not only emotional irritability but also muscular irritability and cramps. Calcium can be taken at night along with magnesium to calm the mood and induce a restful sleep. Women with menopause-related anxiety, mood swings, and fatigue may also find calcium supplementation useful. It has the added benefit of helping prevent bone loss, or osteoporosis, because calcium is a major structural component of bone.

Like magnesium and potassium, calcium is essential in the maintenance of regular heartbeat and the healthy transmission of impulses through the nerves. It may also help reduce blood pressure and regulate cholesterol levels; it is essential for blood clotting. Good sources of calcium include green leafy vegetables, salmon (with bones), nuts and seeds, tofu, and blackstrap molasses.

Iodine. This mineral is necessary to prevent fatigue caused by low thyroid function. Iodine, along with the amino acid tyrosine, is necessary for the production of the thyroid hormone thyroxin. Without adequate thyroid hormone women may suffer from excessive fatigue, excess weight, constipation, and other symptoms of a slowed metabolism. Iodine deficiency has also been linked to breast disease. Only trace amounts of iodine are needed to maintain its important metabolic effects. Good food sources include fish and shellfish, sea vegetables such as kelp and dulse, and garlic.

Essential Fatty Acids for Chronic Fatigue

Essential fatty acids are very important nutrients for women with fatigue and play an important role in maintaining optimal health. Essential fatty acids consist of two types of special fats or oils, called linoleic acid (Omega-6 family) and linolenic acid (Omega-3 family). Because your body cannot make these fats, you must supply them daily via foods or supplements. Though these essential fatty acids supply stored energy in the form of calories, they also perform many other important functions in the body. Essential fatty acids are important components of the membrane structure of all the body's cells. They are also required for normal development and function of the brain, eyes, inner ear, adrenal glands, and reproductive tract. The essential oils are also necessary for the synthesis of prostaglandins type I and III, which are hormonelike chemicals that help decrease the risk of heart disease by regulating blood pressure and platelet stickiness. Prostaglandins type I and II help reduce fatigue through their role in preventing a number of health-care problems: they decrease inflammation, boost immune function, decrease menstrual cramps, and help to reduce PMS symptoms. One essential fat— evening primrose oil—has been tested in the United States and England for its beneficial effects on PMS and menstrual cramps.

Essential oils are particularly important to menopausal women because deficiency of these oils is responsible in part for the drying of skin, hair, vaginal tissues, and other mucous membranes that occurs with menopause. Along with vitamin E, which also benefits the skin and vaginal tissues, I have used essential oils extensively in my nutritional program for women. Essential fatty acids are important in treating immune problems such as candida infections, allergies, and CFS, which worsen fatigue in millions of women.

The best sources of linoleic and linolenic acids are flax seeds and pumpkin seeds. Both the seeds and their pressed oils should be used absolutely fresh and unspoiled. Because these oils become rancid very easily when exposed to light and air (oxygen), they need to be packed in special opaque containers and kept in the refrigerator. Essential oils should never be heated or used in cooking because heat affects their special chemical properties. Instead, add these oils as a flavoring to foods that are already cooked. Fresh flax seed oil is my special favorite. Good quality flax seed oil is available in health food stores or through *The LIFECYCLES Center*. Flax seed oil is golden, rich, and delicious. It is extremely high in linoleic and linolenic acids, which comprise approximately 80 percent of its total content. Pumpkin seed oil has a deep green color and spicy flavor. It is probably more difficult to find than flax seed oil. Fresh raw pumpkin seeds are a good source of this oil. They can be purchased from many health food stores. Both flax seed oil and pumpkin seed oil can also be taken in capsule form.

Linolenic acid (Omega-3 family) is also found in abundance in fish oils. The best sources are cold-water, high-fat fish such as salmon, tuna, rainbow trout, mackerel, and eel. Linoleic acid (Omega-6 family) is found in seeds and seed oils. Good sources include safflower oil, sunflower oil, corn oil, sesame seed oil, and wheat germ oil. Many women prefer to use raw fresh sesame seeds, sunflower seeds, and wheat germ to obtain the oils. The average healthy adult requires only four teaspoons per day of essential oils. However, women with chronic fatigue, who may have a real deficiency of these oils, need up to two or three tablespoons per day until their symptoms improve. Occasionally, these oils may cause diarrhea; if this occurs, use only one teaspoon per day. Women with acne and very oily skin should use them cautiously. For optimal results, be sure to use these oils along with vitamin E.

Herbs for Chronic Fatigue

Many herbs can help relieve the symptoms and treat the causes of chronic fatigue. I have used fatigue-relieving herbs in my practice for many years and many women have found them to be effective remedies. I use them as a form of extended nutrition. They can balance and expand the diet while optimizing nutritional intake. Some herbs provide an additional source of essential nutrients that help relax tension and ease anxiety. Other herbs have mild anti-infective and hormonal properties in addition to their nutritional content; these help to combat fatigue-causing viruses and fungi, as well as provide support for the endocrine system with a minimum of side effects. In this section, I describe many specific herbs useful for relief of chronic fatigue and related problems.

Chronic Fatigue and Depression. For women with fatigue and depression, herbs such as oat straw, ginger, ginkgo biloba, licorice root, dandelion root, and Siberian ginseng (eleutherococcus) may have a stimulatory effect, improving energy and vitality. Women who use these herbs may note an increased ability to handle stress, as well as improved physical and mental capabilities.

Some of the salutary effects may be due to the high levels of essential nutrients captured in herbs. For example, dandelion root contains magnesium, potassium, and vitamin E, while ginkgo contains high levels of bioflavonoids. These essential nutrients help relieve fatigue, depression, PMS, and hot flashes, and they increase resistance to infections.

Siberian ginseng, ginger, and licorice root have been important traditional medicines in China and other countries for thousands of years. They have been reputed to increase longevity and decrease fatigue and weakness. These herbs have been found to boost immunity and to strengthen the cardiovascular system. The bioflavonoids contained in ginkgo are extremely powerful antioxidants and help to combat fatigue by improving circulation to the brain. They also appear to have a strong affinity for the adrenal and thyroid gland and may help to boost function in these essential glands. Oat straw has been used to relieve fatigue and weakness, especially when there is an emotional component. One note of caution: Licorice root should be used carefully and only in small amounts because, over time, it can cause potassium loss.

In modern China, Japan, and other countries, there has been much interest in the pharmacological effects of these traditional herbs. Scientific studies are corroborating the medicinal effects of these plants.

Anxiety, Irritability, and Insomnia. Women suffering from anxiety, irritability and insomnia often have a worsening of their fatigue symptoms because of emotional stress and sleep deprivation. Luckily, a number of herbal remedies relieve such symptoms. Herbs such as passionflower (passiflora) and valerian root have a calming and restful effect on the central nervous system.

Passionflower has been found to elevate levels of the neurotransmitter serotonin. Serotonin is synthesized from tryptophan, an essential amino acid that has been found in numerous medical studies to initiate sleep and decrease awakening. Valerian root has been used extensively in traditional herbology as a sleep inducer. It is used widely in Europe as an effective treatment for insomnia. Research studies have confirmed both the sedative effect of valerian root and its effectiveness as a treatment for insomnia. For women with insomnia, valerian root can be a real blessing. I have used it with patients for the past 18 years and noted much symptom relief. Other effective herbal treatments include chamomile, hops, catnip, and peppermint teas. I have used them all in my practice and many pleased patients have commented on their effectiveness.

Chronic Fatigue Syndrome, Candida Infections, and Allergies. Women with fatigue symptoms caused by severe immune dysfunction may initially have difficulty using any herbs at all because their bodies are too weak. In cases of severe fatigue, I often start the patient on aloe vera and peppermint. Most women can tolerate these two supportive and soothing herbs. You can take aloe vera internally as a juice. Buy the cold-pressed, nonpasteurized brands. You can take peppermint as a tea or, even better, as an oil in capsules or an herbal tincture in water.

Once you are stronger and less fatigued, you may be able to tolerate herbs that can boost your energy and vitality (see information earlier in this section), as well as herbs that help suppress infections from viruses, candida, and other pathogens. One of the best herbs for this purpose is garlic. Garlic contains a chemical called allicin that is a powerful broad spectrum antibiotic. Studies have shown garlic to be effective against fungi such as candida, as well as the fungus that causes athlete's foot and the dangerous fungus that causes serious cryptococcal meningitis. Garlic also kills bacteria and viruses. In addition, garlic protects the cells through its powerful antioxidant effects.

Two other herbs have strong anti-infective properties and can be used to treat pathogens that cause fatigue. The first is echinacea, a powerful immune stimulant herb. Echinacea helps fight infections by promoting interferon production, as well as activation of the T-lymphocytes (natural killer cells) and neutrophils (the cells that kill bacteria). Native Americans traditionally used this plant as a medicinal agent. I have used echinacea often with patients and have been pleased with its powerful anti-infective properties. The second herb, goldenseal, is also an excellent immune stimulant. Goldenseal contains a high level of chemical called berberine. Berberine activates macrophages (cells that engulf and destroy bacteria, fungi, and viruses). When used in combination with garlic and echinacea, goldenseal is an effective tool for suppressing infections.

Menopause, PMS, and Hypothyroidism. Many plants are good sources of estrogen, the hormone that helps control hot flashes in menopausal women. Blueberries, blackberries, huckleberries, and citrus fruit contain bioflavonoids. Bioflavonoids have weak estrogenic activity (1/50,000 the strength of estrogen), but are very effective in controlling such common menopausal symptoms as hot flashes, anxiety, irritability, and fatigue. Plants containing bioflavonoids may be particularly useful for women who cannot take normal supplements because of their concern about the possible strong side effects of the prescription hormones (increased risk of stroke, cancer, etc.). Other plant sources of estrogen and progesterone used in traditional herbology include Dong Quai, black cohosh, blue cohosh, unicorn root, false unicorn root, fennel, anise, sarsaparilla, and wild yam root. The hormonal activities of these plants have been validated in a number of interesting research studies.

Women with PMS also benefit from herbs that relieve mood swings and anxiety, such as valerian root or passionflower, and those that directly reduce fatigue and depression, such as ginger root, ginkgo biloba, and dandelion. Ginger also helps relieve the bloating and fluid retention symptoms of PMS, as do dandelion and burdock root, which act as mild diuretics. Iodine-containing plants, including dulse and kelp, help correct low thyroid function. These sea vegetables are also high in trace minerals, so are excellent for general health and well-being. Iodine is used for the production of thyroxin, the thyroid hormone that helps boost metabolism and maintain energy level.

Anemia and Heavy, Irregular Menstrual Bleeding. Plants that contain bioflavonoids help strengthen capillaries and prevent heavy, irregular menstrual bleeding (menorrhagia), a common bleeding pattern in women approaching menopause. Besides controlling hot flashes, bioflavonoids also help to reduce heavy bleeding. Bioflavonoids are found in many fruits and flowers; excellent sources are citrus fruits, cherries, grapes, and hawthorn berries. According to research studies, they have also been found in red clover and in some clover strains in Australia. Many medical studies have demonstrated the usefulness of citrus bioflavonoids in treating a variety of bleeding problems in addition to those related to menopause, including habitual spontaneous abortion and tuberculosis. Herbs such as yellow dock and pau d'arco are useful for anemia because of their high iron content.

How to Use Optimal Nutritional Formulas for Chronic Fatigue

Good dietary habits are crucial for relief of chronic fatigue, but many women must also use nutritional supplements to achieve high levels of certain essential nutrients. This section contains formulas that you can use to treat fatigue related to different causes. I have included both vitamin and mineral formulas and herbal formulas so that you will have the widest range of supplements to choose from. You can put together any of these formulas yourself. Several of these supplement systems are available from The LIFECYCLES Center (see Appendix for specific information).

I recommend that women with chronic fatigue take all supplements cautiously. Start with one-quarter of the daily dose listed in the following formulas. Do not go to a higher dose level unless you are sure you can tolerate the dose you're already using. If you have specific questions about nutritional supplementation, be sure to consult your physician.

Nutritional System for Chronic Fatigue Syndrome, Candida Infections, Allergies, and Depression

Vitamins and Minerals	Maximum Daily Dose
Beta carotene (provitamin A)	10,000 I.U.
Vitamin B complex	
B_1 (thiamine)	50 mg
B_2 (riboflavin)	75 mg
B_3 (niacinamide)	200 mg
B_5 (pantothenic acid)	200 mg
B_6 (pyridoxine)	75 mg
B_{12} (cyanocobalamin)	100 mcg
Folic acid	400 mcg
Biotin	400 mcg
Choline	700 mg
Inositol	500 mg
PABA (para-aminobenzoic acid)	50 mg
Vitamin C	2000 mg
Vitamin D	200 I.U.
Vitamin E	400 I.U.
Calcium aspartate	1200 mg
Magnesium aspartate	700 mg
Potassium aspartate	200 mg
Iron	18 mg
Chromium	150 mcg
Manganese	20 mg
Selenium	50 mcg
Zinc	15 mg
Copper	2 mg
Iodine	150 mcg

Dosage: Take one-quarter to full amount of the above nutrients on a daily basis. Begin this formula with the lowest dose of each nutrient and increase the dose slowly and gradually to the recommended maximum, depending on how you are feeling.

Herbal Tinctures	Maximum Daily Dose
Ginkgo biloba	2 droppersful
Ginger root	2 droppersful
Burdock root	2 droppersful
Dandelion root	2 droppersful
Licorice root	1/2 dropperful

Dosage: Take one-quarter to full amount of the above nutrients on a daily basis. Begin this formula with the lowest dose of each nutrient and increase the dose slowly and gradually to the recommended maximum, depending on how you are feeling.

Optimal Nutritional Supplementation for PMS and Hypothyroidism

Vitamins and Minerals	Maximum Daily Dose
Beta carotene (provitamin A)	15,000 I.U.
Vitamin B complex	
B_1 (thiamine)	50 mg
B_2 (riboflavin)	50 mg
B_3 (niacinamide)	50 mg
B_5 (pantothenic acid)	50 mg
B_6 (pyridoxine HCl)	300 mcg
B_{12} (cyanocobalamin)	50 mcg
Folic acid	200 mcg
Biotin	30 mcg
Choline bitartrate	500 mg
Inositol	500 mg
PABA (para-aminobenzoic acid)	50 mg
Vitamin C	1000 mg
Vitamin D (cholecalciferol)	100 I.U.
Vitamin E	600 I.U.
Calcium (amino acid chelate)	150 mg
Magnesium	300 mg
Iodine	150 mcg

Vitamins and Minerals	Maximum Daily Dose
Iron (amino acid chelate)	15 mg
Copper	0.5 mg
Zinc	25 mg
Manganese	10 mg
Potassium	100 mg
Selenium	25 mcg
Chromium	100 mcg

Dosage: Take one-quarter to full amount of the above nutrients on a daily basis. Begin this formula with the lowest dose of each nutrient and increase the dose slowly and gradually to the recommended maximum, depending on how you are feeling.

Herbs (as capsules)	Maximum Daily Dose
Burdock	210 mg
Sarsaparilla	210 mg
Ginger	70 mg

Dosage: Take one to two capsules per day.

Optimal Nutritional Supplementation for Fatigue Related to Menopause

Vitamins and Minerals	Maximum Daily Dose
Beta carotene	5000 I.U.
Vitamin A	5000 I.U.
Vitamin D	400 I.U.
Vitamin E (d-alpha tocopheryl acetate)	800 I.U.
Vitamin C	1000 mg
Bioflavonoids	800 mg
Rutin	200 mg
Vitamin B_1	50 mg
Vitamin B_2	50 mg
Niacin (as niacinamide)	50 mg

Vitamins and Minerals	Maximum Daily Dose
Vitamin B_6	30 mg
Vitamin B_{12}	50 mcg
Folic acid	400 mcg
Biotin	200 mcg
Pantothenic acid	50 mg
Choline	50 mg
Inositol	50 mg
PABA (para-aminobenzoic acid)	50 mg
Calcium (calcium citrate)	1200 mg
Magnesium	320 mg
Iodine	150 mcg
Iron (ferrous fumarate)	27 mg
Copper	2 mg
Zinc	15 mg
Manganese	10 mg
Potassium (potassium aspartate)	100 mg
Selenium	25 mcg
Chromium	100 mcg
Bromelain	100 mg
Papain	65 mg
Boron	3 mg

Dosage: Women with mild to moderate menopause symptoms can use the formula at half strength. Women with severe symptoms should use the full strength.

Herbs (as capsules)	Maximum Daily Dose
Fennel	100 mg
Anise	100 mg
Blessed thistle	100 mg
False unicorn root	100 mg
Blue cohosh	100 mg

Dosage: Take one to two capsules per day.

Optimal Nutritional Supplementation for Anemia

Vitamins and Minerals	Maximum Daily Dose
Iron	27 mg
Vitamin C	250 mg
Vitamin E (natural d-alpha)	30 I.U.
Vitamin B_1 (thiamine)	7.5 mg
Vitamin B_2 (riboflavin)	7.5 mg
Vitamin B_6 (pyridoxine)	30 mg
Vitamin B_5 (pantothenic acid)	50 mg
Vitamin B_3 (niacinamide)	10 mg
Vitamin B_{12} (cyanocobalamin)	250 mcg
Folic acid	400 mcg
Biotin	100 mcg
Choline bitartrate	5 mg
Inositol	5 mg
PABA (para-aminobenzoic acid)	5 mg
Zinc	1.5 mg
Copper	250 mcg
Betaine HCL	10 mg

Herbs	Maximum Daily Dose
Chlorophyll	2 droppersful
Yellow dock	2 droppersful
Pau d'arco	2 droppersful
Licorice root	1/2 dropperful
Red clover	1 dropperful

Dosage: Take one-quarter to full amount of the above nutrients on a daily basis. Begin this formula with the lowest dose of each nutrient and increase the dose slowly and gradually to the recommended maximum, depending on how you are feeling.

Food Sources of Vitamin A

Vegetables	Fruits	Meat, Poultry, Seafood
Carrots	Apricots	Crab
Carrot juice	Avocado	Halibut
Collard greens	Cantaloupe	Liver—all types
Dandelion greens	Mangoes	Mackerel
Green onion	Papaya	Salmon
Kale	Peaches	Swordfish
Parsley	Persimmons	
Spinach		
Sweet potatoes		
Turnip greens		
Winter squash		

Food Sources of Vitamin B Complex (including folic acid)

Vegetables and Legumes	Vegetables and Legumes	Meat, Poultry, Seafood
Alfalfa	Green peas	Egg yolks*
Artichokes	Kale	Liver*
Asparagus	Leeks	
Beets	Lentils	*Grains*
Broccoli	Lima beans	Barley
Brussels sprouts	Onions	Bran
Cabbage	Pinto beans	Brown rice
Cauliflower	Romaine lettuce	Corn
Corn	Soybeans	Millet
Garbanzo beans		Rice bran
Green beans		Wheat
		Wheat germ

Eggs and meat should be from organic range-fed stock fed on pesticide-free food.

Sweeteners
Black-strap molasses

Food Sources of Vitamin B$_6$

Grains	Vegetables	Meat, Poultry, Seafood
Brown rice	Asparagus	Chicken
Buckwheat flour	Beet greens	Salmon
Rice bran	Broccoli	Shrimp
Rice polishings	Brussels sprouts	Tuna
Rye flour	Cauliflower	
Wheat germ	Green peas	Nuts and seeds
Whole wheat flour	Leeks	Sunflower seeds
	Sweet potatoes	

Food sources of Vitamin B$_{12}$

Fish
Eggs*
Liver*

Food Sources of Vitamin C

Fruits	Vegetables	Meat, Poultry, Seafood
Blackberries	Asparagus	Liver—all types
Black currants	Black-eyed peas	Pheasant
Cantaloupe	Broccoli	Quail
Elderberries	Brussels sprouts	Salmon
Grapefruit	Cabbage	
Grapefruit juice	Cauliflower	
Guavas	Collards	
Kiwi fruit	Green onions	
Mangoes	Green peas	
Oranges	Kale	
Orange juice	Kohlrabi	
Pineapple	Parsley	
Raspberries	Potatoes	
Strawberries	Rutabaga	
Tangerines	Sweet pepper	
	Sweet potatoes	
	Tomatoes	
	Turnips	

Food Sources of Iron (listed from best to good)

Grains
Bran cereal (All-Bran)
Millet, dry
Wheat germ
Pasta, whole wheat
Bran muffin
Pumpernickel bread
Oak flakes
Shredded wheat
Whole wheat bread
Rye bread
Wheat bran
Pearl barley
White rice

Fruits
Prune juice
Figs
Raisins
Prunes, dried
Avocado
Apple juice
Dates, dried
Blackberries
Pineapple
Grape juice
Apricots, fresh
Cantaloupe
Strawberries
Cherries

Legumes
Black beans
Pinto beans
Garbanzo beans
Soybeans
Kidney beans
Lima beans
Lentils
Split peas
Black-eyed peas
Tofu

Meat, Poultry, Seafood
Calf's liver
Beef liver
Chicken liver
Oysters
Trout
Clams
Scallops
Sardines
Shrimp
Chicken
Haddock
Cod
Salmon

Vegetables
Brussels sprouts
Spinach
Broccoli
Sweet potatoes

Vegetables (cont.)
Dandelion greens
Green beans
Corn
Leeks
Kale
Swiss chard
Beets
Beet greens
Mushrooms
Green peas
Parsnips
Carrots
Mustard greens
Green pepper
Lettuce
Turnips
Asparagus
Collards
Cauliflower
Zucchini
Winter squash
Red cabbage

Nuts and Seeds
Sesame seeds
Sunflower seeds
Pistachios
Pecans
Sesame butter
Almonds
Hazelnuts (filberts)
Walnuts

Food Sources of Zinc

Grains
Barley
Brown rice
Buckwheat
Corn
Cornmeal
Millet
Oatmeal
Rice bran
Rye bread
Wheat bran
Wheat germ
Wheat berries
Whole wheat bread
Whole wheat flour

Vegetables and Legumes
Black-eyed peas
Cabbage
Carrots
Garbanzo beans
Green peas
Lentils
Lettuce
Lima beans
Onions
Soy flour
Soy meal
Soy protein

Fruits
Apples
Peaches

Meat, Poultry, Seafood
Chicken
Oysters

Food Sources of Calcium

Vegetables and Legumes

Artichoke
Black beans
Black-eyed peas
Beet greens
Broccoli
Brussels sprouts
Cabbage
Collards
Eggplant
Garbanzo beans
Green beans
Green onions
Kale
Kidney beans
Leeks
Lentils
Parsley
Parsnips
Pinto beans
Rutabaga
Soybeans
Spinach
Turnips
Watercress

Meat, Poultry, Seafood

Abalone
Beef
Bluefish
Carp
Crab
Haddock
Herring
Lamb
Lobster
Oysters
Perch
Salmon
Shrimp
Venison

Fruits

Blackberries
Black currants
Boysenberries
Oranges
Pineapple juice
Prunes
Raisins
Rhubarb
Tangerine juice

Grains

Bran
Brown rice
Bulgar wheat
Millet

Food Sources of Magnesium

Vegetables and Legumes	Nuts and Seeds	Meat, Poultry, Seafood
Artichokes	Almonds	Beef
Black-eyed peas	Brazil nuts	Carp
Carrot juice	Hazelnuts	Chicken
Corn	Peanuts	Clams
Green peas	Pistachios	Cod
Leeks	Pumpkin seeds	Crab
Lima beans	Sesame seeds	Duck
Okra	Walnuts	Haddock
Parsnips		Herring
Potatoes	**Fruits**	Lamb
Soybean sprouts	Avocado	Mackerel
Spinach	Bananas	Oysters
Squash	Grapefruit juice	Salmon
Yams	Papayas	Shrimp
	Pineapple juice	Snapper
Grains	Prunes	Turkey
Brown rice	Raisins	
Millet		
Wild rice		

Suggested Reading

Castleman, M. *The Healing Herbs.* Emmaus, PA: Rodale Press, 1991.

Crook, W., M.D. *Chronic Fatigue Syndrome and the Yeast Connection.* Jackson, TN: Professional Books, 1992.

Crook, W., M.D. *The Yeast Connection.* Jackson, TN: Professional Books, 1983.

Erasmus, U. *Fats and Oils.* Burnaby, BC, Canada: Alive Books, 1986.

Gittleman, A. L. *Supernutrition for Women.* New York: Bantam Books, 1991.

Hasslering, B., S. Greenwood, M.D., and M. Castleman. *The Medical Self-Care Book of Women's Health.* New York: Doubleday, 1987.

Hogladaroom, G., R. McCorkle, and N. Woods. *The Complete Book of Women's Health.* Englewood Cliffs, NJ: Prentice-Hall, 1982.

Kirschmann, J., and L. Dunne. *Nutrition Almanac.* New York: McGraw-Hill, 1984.

Kutsky, R. *Vitamins and Hormones.* New York: Van Nostrand Reinhold, 1973.

Lambert-Lagace, L. *The Nutrition Challenge for Women.* Palo Alto, CA: Bull Publishing, 1990.

Lark, S., M.D. *Anemia and Heavy Menstrual Flow: A Self-Help Program.* Los Altos, CA: Westchester Publishing, 1993.

Lark, S., M.D. *Menopause Self-Help Book.* Berkeley, CA: Celestial Arts, 1990.

Lark, S., M.D. *Menstrual Cramps: A Self-Help Program.* Los Altos, CA: Westchester Publishing, 1993.

Lark, S., M.D. *Premenstrual Syndrome Self-Help Book.* Berkeley, CA: Celestial Arts, 1984.

Mowrey, D., Ph.D. *The Scientific Validation of Herbal Medicine.* New Canaan, CT: Keats Publishing, 1986.

Murray, M., N.D. *The 21st Century Herbal.* Bellevue, WA: Vita-Line, Inc., 1992.

Padus, E. *The Woman's Encyclopedia of Health and Natural Healing.* Emmaus, PA: Rodale Press, 1981.

Reuben, C., and J. Priestly, M.D. *Essential Supplements for Women*. New York: Perigree Books, 1988.

Trowbridge, J., M.D., and M. Walker, D.M.P. *The Yeast Syndrome*. New York: Bantam Books, 1988.

Articles

Abou-Saleh, M. T., and A. Coopen. The biology of folate in depression: Implications for nutritional hypotheses of the psychoses. *Journal of Psychiatric Research* 1986; 20(2):91–101.

Abraham, G. E. Nutritional factors in the etiology of the premenstrual tension syndromes. *Journal of Reproductive Medicine* 1983; 28(7):446-64.

Abraham, G. E. Premenstrual tension. *Problems in Obstetrics & Gynecology* 3(12):1–39.

Abraham, G. E., and J. T. Hargrove. Effect of vitamin B_6 on premenstrual symptomatology in women with premenstrual tension syndrome: A double-blind cross-over study. *Infertility* 1980; 3:155–165.

Adetumbi, M. A., and B. H. Lau. Allium sativum (garlic): A natural antibiotic. *Medical Hypotheses* 1983; 12(3):227–37.

Amelia, M., et al. Inhibition of mast cell histamine release by flavonoids and bioflavonoids. *Planta Medica* 1985; 51:16–20.

Amer, M., M. Taha, and Z. Tosson. The effect of aqueous garlic extract on the growth of dermatophytes. *International Journal of Dermatology* 1980; 19:285.

Axelrod A. E., and A. C. Trakatellis. Relationship of pyridoxine to immunological phenomena. *Vitamins and Hormones* 1964; 22:591–607.

Baehner, R. I., and L. A. Boxer. Role of membrane vitamin E and cytoplasmic glutathione in the regulation of phagocytic functions of neutrophils and monocytes. *American Journal of Pediatric Hematology and Oncology* 1979; 1(1):71–76.

Baird, I. M., et al. The effects of ascorbic acid and flavonoids on the occurrence of symptoms normally associated with the common cold. *American Journal of Clinical Nutrition* 1979; 32:1686–90.

Banki, C. M., et al. Cerebrospinal fluid magnesium and calcium related to amine metabolites, diagnosis and suicide attempts. *Biological Psychiatry* 1985; 20:163–71.

Barr, W. Pyridoxine supplements in the premenstrual syndrome. *Practitioner* 1984; 228:425–27.

Beisel, W. R. Single nutrients and immunity. *American Journal of Clinical Nutrition* 1982; 35:417–68 (suppl.).

Bondestam, M., et al. Subclinical trace element deficiency in children with undue susceptibility to infections. *Acta Paediatrica Scandinavica* 1985; 74(4):515–20.

Brush, M. G., and M. Perry. Pyridoxine and the premenstrual syndrome. *Lancet* 1985; 1:1339.

Carney, M. W., et al. Thiamine, riboflavin and pyridoxine deficiency in psychiatric in-patients. *British Journal of Psychiatry* 1982; 141:271–72.

Chandra, R. K. Trace element regulation of immunity and infection. *Journal of the American College of Nutrition* 1985; 4(1):5–16.

Cheng, E. W., et al. Estrogenic activity of some naturally occurring isoflavones. *Annals of New York Academy of Sciences* 1955; 61(30):652.

Cheraskin, E., et al. Daily vitamin C consumption and fatigability. *Journal of the American Geriatric Society* 1976; 24(3):136–37.

Christy, C. J. Vitamin E in menopause. *American Journal of Obstetrics and Gynecology* 1945; 50:84.

Clemetson, C. A. Histamine and ascorbic acid in human blood. *Journal of Nutrition* 1980; 110(4):662–68.

Clemetson, C. A., et al. Capillary strength and the menstrual cycle. *New York Academy of Science* 1962; 93(7):277.

Cohen, J. D., and H. W. Rubin. Functional menorrhagia: treatment with bioflavonoids and vitamin C. *Current Therapeutic Research* 1960; 2(11):539.

Das, K. C., and V. Herbert. The lymphocyte as a marker of past nutritional status: Persistence of abnormal lymphocyte deoxyuridine (uD) suppression test and chromosomes in patients with past deficiency of folate and vitamin B_{12}. *British Journal of Hematology* 1978; 38:219–33.

Das, U. N. Antibiotic-like action of essential fatty acids. *Journal of Canadian Medical Association* 1985; 132:1350.

Duchateau, J., et al. Influence of oral zinc supplementation on the lymphocyte response to mitogens of normal subjects. *American Journal of Clinical Nutrition* 1981; 34:88–93.

Ellis, F. R., and S. Nasser. A pilot study of vitamin B_{12} in the treatment of tiredness. *British Journal of Nutrition* 1973; 30:277–83.

Finkler, R. S. The effect of vitamin E in the menopause. *Journal of Clinical Endocrinology and Metabolism* 1949; 9:89–94.

Folkers, K., et al. Biochemical evidence for a deficiency of vitamin B_6 in subjects reacting to monosodium-L-glutamate by the Chinese restaurant syndrome. *Biochemical and Biophysical Research Communication* 1981; 100:972–77.

Foreman, J. C. Editorial: Mast cells and the actions of flavonoids. *Journal of Allergy and Clinical Immunology* 1984; 73:769–74.

Formica, P. E. The housewife syndrome: Treatment with potassium and magnesium salts of aspartic acid. *Current Therapeutic Research* March 1962; 4:98.

Frizel, D., et al. Plasma calcium and magnesium in depression. *British Journal of Psychiatry* 1969; 115:1375–77.

Gaby, A. R. Aspartic acid salts and fatigue. *Current Nutritional Therapeutics* November 1982.

Gardner, G. W., et al. Physical work capacity and metabolic stress in subjects with iron deficiency anemia. *American Journal of Clinical Nutrition* 1977; 30(6):910–17.

Ghadirian, A. M., et al. Folic acid deficiency and depression. *Psychosomatics* 1980; 21(11): 926–29.

Gozan, H. A. The use of vitamin E in treatment of the menopause. *New York State Medical Journal* 1952; 1289–91.

Hines, J. D, and D. Love. Abnormal vitamin B_6 metabolism in sideroblastic anemia: Effect of pyridoxal phosphate therapy. *Clinical Research* 1975; 23:403A.

Hines, J. D., and J. W. Harris. Pyridoxine-responsive anemia: Description of three patients with megaloblastic erythopoiesis. *American Journal of Clinical Nutrition* 1964; 14:137–46.

Hodges, R. E., et al. Hematopoietic studies in vitamin A deficiency. *American Journal of Clinical Nutrition* 1978; 31:876–85.

Horrobin, D. F. Essential fatty acid and prostaglandin metabolism in Sjogren's Syndrome, systemic sclerosis and rheumatoid arthritis. *Scandinavian Journal of Rheumatology Supplement* 1980; 61:242.

Horrobin, D. F. Essential fatty acids in clinical dermatology. *Journal of the American Academy of Dermatology* 1987; 20(6):1045.

Horrobin, D. F. The regulation of prostaglandin biosynthesis by the manipulation of essential fatty acid metabolism. *Revue of Pure and Applied Pharmacological Science* Oct/Dec 1980; 4(4):339.

Horrobin, D. F. The role of essential fatty acids and prostaglandins in the premenstrual syndrome. *Journal of Reproductive Medicine* 1983; 28(7):465.

Hunt, J. R., et al. Ascorbic acid: Effect on ongoing iron absorption and status in iron-depleted young women. *American Journal of Clinical Nutrition* 1990; 51:649–55.

Judge, T. G., and N. R. Cowan. Dietary potassium intake and grip strength in older people. *Gerontologia Clinica* 1971; 13:221–26.

Kaplan, S. S., and R. E. Basford. Effect of vitamin B_{12} and folic acid deficiencies on neutrophil function. *Blood* 1976; 47:801–5.

Laul, T. N., et al. Antiviral effect of flavonoids on human viruses. *Journal of Medical Virology* 1985; 15:71–79.

Kavinoky, N. R. Vitamin E and the control of climacteric symptoms. *Annals of Western Medicine and Surgery* 1950; 4(1):27–32.

Krotkiewski, M., et al. Zinc and muscle strength endurance. *Acta Physiologica Scandinavica* 1982; 116(3):309–11.

Lane, M., and C. P. Alfrey, Jr. The anemia of human riboflavin deficiency. *Blood* 1965; 25(4):432–42.

Leitner, Z. A., and I. C. Church. Nutritional studies in a mental hospital. *Lancet* 1956; 1:565–67.

Lightgow, P. M., and W. M. Politzer. Vitamin A in the treatment of menorrhagia. *Journal of South African Medicine* 1977; 51:191.

Leonard, P. J., and M. S. Losowsky. Effect of alpha-tocopherol administration on red cell survival in vitamin E-deficient human subjects. *American Journal of Clinical Nutrition* 1971; 24:388–93.

Ludvigsson, J., et al. Vitamin C as a preventive medicine against common colds in children. *Scandinavian Journal of Infectious Disease* 1977; 9(2):91–98.

Manku, M. S., et al. Reduced levels of prostaglandin precursors in the blood of atopic patients: Defective delta-6-desaturase function as a biochemical basis for atopy. *Prostaglandins Leukotrienes and Medicine* 1982; 9(6):615–28.

Meija, L., and F. Chew. Hematologic effect on supplementing anemic children with vitamin A alone and in combination with iron. *American Journal of Clinical Nutrition* 1988; 48:595–600.

Middleton, E., Jr., and G. Drzewiecki. Flavonoid inhibition of human basophil histamine release stimulated by various germs. *Biochemistry Pharmacology* 1984; 33(21):3333.

Miller, J. Z., et al. Therapeutic effect of vitamin C. A co-twin control study. *Journal of the American Medical Association* 1977; 237(3):248–51.

Milner, G. Ascorbic acid in chronic psychiatric patients: A controlled trial. *British Journal of Psychiatry* 1963; 109:294–99.

Monsen, E. R. Ascorbic acid: An enhancing factor in iron absorption in nutritional bioavailability of iron. *American Chemical Society* 1982; 85–95.

Pearce, F., et al. Mucosal mast cells, Ill. Effect of quercetin and other flavonoids on antigen induced histamine secretion from rat intestinal mast cells. *Journal of Allergy and Clinical Immunology* 1984; 73:819–23.

Pearse, H. A., and J. D. Trisler. A rational approach to the treatment of habitual abortion and menometorrhagia. *Clinical Medicine* 1957; 9:1081.

Pitt, H. A., and A. M. Costrini. Vitamin C prophylaxis in Marine recruits. *Journal of the American Medical Association* March 1979; 241:908–11.

Pope, G. S., et al. Isolation of an oestrogenic isoflavone (biochanin A) from red clover. *Chemistry and Industry* 1953; 10:1042.

Prasad, G., and V. D. Sharma. Efficacy of garlic (Allium sativum) treatment against experimental Candidiasis in chicks. *Journal of British Veterinary Medicine* 1980; 136:448.

Rabinowitz, P. S., and H. S. Nelson. The effect of ascorbic acid on cutaneous and nasal response to histamine and allergen. *Journal of Allergy and Clinical Immunology* 1982; 69(6):484–88.

Richardson, J. H., and M. Chenman. The effect of B_6 on muscle fatigue. *Journal of Sports Medicine and Physical Fitness* 1981; 21(2):119–21.

Rosen, H., et al. Effects of the potassium and magnesium salts of aspartic acid on metabolic exhaustion. *Journal of Pharmaceutical Science* 1962; 51:592.

Salvin, S. B., and B. S. Rabin. Resistance and susceptibility to infection in inbred murine strains. IV. Effects of dietary zinc. *Cellular Immunology* 1984; 87(2):546–52.

Schwerdt, P. R., and C. E. Schwerdt. Effect of ascorbic acid on rhinovirus replication in WI-38 cells. *Proceedings of the Society of Biological Medicine* 1975; 148:1237.

Simon, S. W. Vitamin B_{12} therapy in allergy and chronic dermatoses. *Journal of Allergy* 1951; 2:183–85.

Smith, C. J. Non-hormonal control of vaso-motor flushing in menopausal patients. *Chicago Medicine* March 1964.

Stewart, J. W., et al. Low B_6 levels in depressed outpatients. *Biological Psychiatry* 1984; 19(4):613–16.

Taylor, F. A. Habitual abortion: Therapeutic evaluation of citrus bioflavonoids. *Western Journal of Surgical Obstetrics and Gynecology* 1956; 5:280.

Taymor, M. L., et al. The etiological role of chronic iron deficiency in production of menorrhagia. *Journal of the American Medical Association* 1964; 187:323.

Taymor, M. L., et al. Menorrhagia due to chronic iron deficiency. *Obstetrics and Gynecology* 1960; 16:571.

van der Beek, E. J. Vitamins and endurance training: Food for running or faddish claims? *Sports Medicine* 1985; 2(3):175–97.

Webb, W. L., and M. Gehi. Electrolyte and fluid imbalance: Neuropsychiatric manifestations. *Psychosomatics* 1981; 22(3):199–203.

Zucker, D. K., et al. B_{12} deficiency and psychiatric disorders: Case report and literature review. *Biological Psychiatry* 1981; 16:197–205.

7

Stress Reduction for Relief of Chronic Fatigue

Stress is a major trigger for the symptoms of chronic fatigue. Women who are already tired because of an imbalance in body chemistry and physiology may find that the addition of stress and tension in their everyday lives can increase their fatigue to a serious and debilitating level. Women with chronic fatigue often need to develop more effective ways of dealing with day-to-day stresses. The minor everyday stresses that women with normal energy levels handle easily can be overwhelming for women whose energy reserves are low. Moreover, significant lifestyle changes—death of a loved one, divorce, job loss, financial problems, major changes in personal relationships—can be almost impossible to handle when a woman is chronically fatigued. Being unable to cope with stress effectively can also damage a woman's self-esteem and self-confidence. In addition to the physical symptoms, a woman with chronic fatigue may feel a decreasing sense of self-worth as her ability to handle her usual range of activities diminishes. This can often lead to deepening depression and a tendency to become more isolated as the chronic fatigue symptoms progress.

Since the life stresses themselves don't necessarily change, how a woman copes with them can really make the difference.

Many of my women patients feel that stress is contributing to their fatigue level; they are looking for ways to handle their stress more effectively. Even women who are completely happy with their professional and personal lives feel that effective stress management would help reduce fatigue.

How Stress Tires the Body

Your reaction to stress is partly determined by how sensitive your autonomic nervous system is. The autonomic nervous system regulates the bodily functions that we are usually unaware of—pulse rate, respiration, muscle tension, glandular function, and circulation of the blood. It is divided into two parts that oppose and complement each other, called the sympathetic and parasympathetic nervous systems. For example, if fear or excitement speeds up the heart rate too much, the parasympathetic nervous system acts as a control circuit and slows down the heart rate. If the heart slows down too much, then the sympathetic nervous system speeds it up. Thus, the parasympathetic and sympathetic nervous systems have the job of controlling the upper and lower limits of your physiology.

Either major or minor lifestyle upsets may cause an overreaction of the sympathetic system in a woman with chronic fatigue because she has little reserve to deal with such stresses. An easily triggered sympathetic nervous system causes your muscles to tense, your blood vessels to constrict, your adrenal glands to pump out hormones, and your heart and pulse rates to speed up so you can react to an emergency. If you have an especially stressful life, your sympathetic nervous system may always be poised to react to a crisis. This puts you in a state of constant tension, sometimes known as "fight or flight." In this mode, you tend to react to small stresses the same way you would react to real emergencies. The energy that accumulates in the body to meet this "emergency" must then be discharged to bring your body back into balance. The end result of the "fight or flight" reaction in women with chronic fatigue is that the repeated process depletes your energy reserves, continuing in a downward spiral that can lead to complete exhaustion. You can break this spiral only by learning to manage stress effectively in a way that protects and even increases your energy level.

Techniques for Relaxation

Many patients have asked me about techniques for coping more effectively with stress. Although I send some women for counseling or psychotherapy, most are looking for practical ways to manage stress on their own. They want to take responsibility for learning to handle their own problems—observing their inadequate methods of dealing with stress, learning new techniques to improve their habits, and then practicing these techniques on a regular basis. I have included relaxation and stress reduction exercises in many of my patient programs. The feedback has been very positive; many patients report an increased sense of well-being from these self-help techniques. They also note an improvement in their physical health. This chapter includes a series of eight stress-reduction exercises that I have developed for women with chronic fatigue. Try them all and decide which ones produce the greatest benefits for you; practice those on a regular basis.

Handling Negative Thoughts and Feelings

Throughout the day your conscious mind may be barraged with thoughts, feelings, and fantasies about your daily life. Many of these thoughts replay unresolved issues of health, finances, or personal relationships that are causing you anxiety and discomfort. A woman with chronic fatigue can find this relentless mental replay of unresolved issues exhausting. It is important to know how to shut off the constant inner dialogue and quiet the mind. The first two exercises require you to sit quietly and engage in a simple repetitive activity. By emptying your mind, you give yourself a rest. Meditation allows you to create a state of deep relaxation, which is very healing to the entire body. Metabolism is slowed, as are physiological functions such as heart rate and blood pressure. Muscle tension decreases. Brain wave patterns shift from the fast beta waves that occur during a normal active day to the slower alpha waves. Alpha waves also appear just before falling asleep or in times of deep relaxation. If you practice these exercises regularly, they can help relieve chronic fatigue by resting your mind and turning off any upsetting thoughts.

Exercise 1: Concentration

Select a small piece of your personal jewelry that you like a great deal. It might be a jeweled pin or a pair of pearl earrings. Focus all your attention on this object as you inhale and exhale slowly and deeply for one to two minutes. While you are doing this exercise, don't let any other thoughts or feelings enter your mind. At the end of this exercise you will probably feel more peaceful and calmer. Any tension or nervousness that you were feeling upon starting the exercise should be diminished.

Exercise 2: Meditation

- Sit or lie in a comfortable position. Allow your arms to rest by your sides. Begin to inhale and exhale slowly and deeply with your eyes closed.

- As you inhale, say the word "one" to yourself, and as you exhale, say the word "two." Draw out the pronunciation of the word so that it lasts for the entire breath: o-o-o-o-n-n-n-n-n-e-e-e-e, t-w-w-w-w-o-o-o-o-o-o. Repeating these words as you breathe will help you to concentrate.

- Focus all your attention on your breathing. Notice your chest and abdomen moving in and out.

- Block out all other feelings and thoughts. If your attention wanders, refocus on your breathing and word repetition.

- Do this exercise for 10 or 15 minutes.

Exercise 3: Release of Muscle Tension and Negative Emotion

This exercise helps you focus on areas in your body that have chronic muscle tension and helps you become aware of how you feel and perceive this tension. Often, habitual emotional patterns cause certain muscle groups to tense and tighten. For example, if a person has difficulty in expressing feelings, the neck muscles may be chronically tense. A person with a lot of repressed anger may have chest pain and tight chest muscles. Blocked emotions cause contracted muscles, which limit movement and energy flow in the body. Muscle tension can be a significant cause of chronic fatigue. This exercise helps release tension and the blocked emotions held in tight muscles.

• Lie in a comfortable position. Allow your arms to rest at your sides, palms down. Inhale and exhale slowly and deeply with your eyes closed.

• Become aware of your feet, ankles, and legs. Notice if these parts of your body have any muscle tension or tightness. If so, how does the tense part of your body feel? Is it viselike, knotted, cold, numb? Do you notice any strong feelings, such as hurt, upset, or anger, in that part of your body? Breathe into that part of your body until you feel it relax. Release any negative emotions with your breathing, continuing until they begin to decrease in intensity and fade.

• Next, move your awareness into your hips, pelvis, and lower back. Note any tension there. Notice any negative feelings located in that part of your body. Breathe into your hips and pelvis until you feel them relax. Release any negative emotions as you breathe in and out.

• Focus on your abdomen and chest. Notice any negative feelings located in this area and let them drop away as you breathe in and out. Continue to release any upsetting feelings located in your abdomen or chest.

- Finally, focus on your head, neck, arms, and hands. Note any tension in this area and release it. With your breathing, release any negative feelings blocked in this area until you can't feel them anymore.

- When you have finished releasing tension throughout the body, continue deep breathing and relaxing for another minute or two. At the end of this exercise, you should feel lighter and more energized.

Visualization

The next three exercises use visualization as a therapeutic method to affect the physical and mental processes of the body; two focus on color, the third on a healthy body. Color therapy, as it applies to human health, has a long and distinguished history. In several studies, scientists exposed subjects to specific colors, either directly through exposure to light therapy, or through changing the color of their environment. Scientific research throughout the world has shown that color therapy can have a profound effect on health and well-being. It can stimulate the endocrine glands, the immune system, and the nervous system, which are weakened in women with chronic fatigue. Visualizing color in a specific part of the body can have a powerful therapeutic effect, too, and can be an effective stress management technique for relief of chronic fatigue.

The first exercise uses the color blue, which provides a calming and relaxing effect. For women with chronic fatigue who are carrying a lot of physical and emotional tension, blue eliminates the "flight or fight" response. (This response stresses the adrenal glands and, over time, leads to exhaustion.) Blue also calms physiological functions such as pulse rate, breathing, and perspiration, and relaxes the mood. It should be used primarily by fatigued women who are chronically tense, anxious, irritable, or carry a lot of muscle tension.

The second exercise uses the color red, which can benefit all women who have fatigue. Red stimulates all the endocrine glands, including the pituitary and adrenal glands. It heightens senses such as smell and taste. Autonomic nervous system function speeds up with increased blood flow and blood pressure; metabolic rate increases, too. Emotionally, red is linked to vitality and high energy states. I often do the red visualization when I am tired and need a pick-me-up.

Exercise 4: Tension Release Through Color

- Sit or lie in a comfortable position, your arms resting at your sides. As you take a deep breath, visualize that the earth below you is filled with the color blue. This blue color extends 50 feet below you into the earth. Now imagine that you are opening up energy centers on the bottom of your feet. As you inhale, visualize the soft blue color filling up your feet. When your feet are completely filled with the color blue, then bring the color up through your ankles, legs, pelvis, and lower back.

- Each time you exhale, see the blue color leaving through your lungs, carrying any tension and stress with it. See the tension dissolve into the air.

- Continue to inhale blue into your abdomen, chest, shoulders, arms, neck, and head. Exhale the blue slowly out of your lungs. Repeat this entire process 5 times and then relax for a few minutes.

Exercise 5: Energizing Through Color

- Sit or lie in a comfortable position, your arms resting easily at your sides. As you take a deep breath, visualize a big balloon above your head filled with a bright red healing energy. Imagine that you pop this balloon so all the bright red energy is released.

- As you inhale, see the bright red color filling up your head. It fills up your brain, your face, and the bones of your skull. Let the bright red color pour in until your head is ready to overflow with color. Then let the red color flow into your neck, shoulders, arms, and chest. As you exhale, breathe the red color out of your lungs, taking any tiredness and fatigue with it. Breathe any feeling of fatigue out of your body.

- As you inhale, continue to bring the bright, energizing red color into your abdomen, pelvis, lower back, legs, and feet until your whole body is filled with red. Exhale the red color out of your lungs, continuing to release any feeling of fatigue. Repeat this process 5 times. At the end of this exercise, you should feel more energized and vibrant, your mental energy more vitalized and clear.

Exercise 6: Visualization for a Healthy Body

When you visualize your body as healthy, strong, and vital, you begin to lay down the mental blueprint for better health. This technique of actually imaging your body the way that you want it to be has been used in the treatment of cancer as well as other serious diseases. This technique was pioneered by Carl Simonton, M.D., a cancer radiation therapist. A number of his patients, after using this technique to stimulate their immune systems and shrink their tumors, saw their diseases go into remission. Here you use the same type of visualization to relieve chronic fatigue.

- Close your eyes and begin to breathe deeply, slowly inhaling and exhaling. Feel your body begin to relax.

- Imagine that you are looking in a mirror. Actually see yourself in your mind's eye. You may be undressed or wearing just a slip or shorts.

- Look at your face; it is full of vibrant energy. Your skin is glowing and healthy looking. Your eyes are bright and clear. Look at your hair; it has a healthy sheen. Your face is confident and smiling. You feel tension-free and in command of yourself. As you see yourself in the mirror, you are pleased with how vibrant and energized you look. You feel you could handle with ease any problems that come along.

- Now look at your entire body. It radiates health and well-being. Look at your breasts, your abdomen, your hips, legs, and feet. You can almost see the energy and vitality running through your entire body. You can actually visualize a current of energy running through every part of your body. Your body looks strong, sturdy, and healthy. You feel optimistic and confident. Your mood is calm and relaxed.

- Now stop visualizing the scene and focus again on deep breathing. After 15 or 20 seconds, open your eyes and continue to relax for a minute or two.

Affirmations

The following two exercises give you healthful affirmations that can be very useful for women with chronic fatigue. When I work with a patient, I always stress the important connection between the mind and body. Your state of health is determined in part by the thousands of mental messages you send yourself each day with your thoughts. To truly heal from any health problem, the mind and body must work together in a positive way. It is not enough to follow a good diet and take the medication that a physician prescribes. When your body believes it is sick, it behaves as if it is sick. For example, if you have a peptic ulcer and your belief is that you can never really get well, the ulcer pain will worsen. If you believe that your arthritis symptoms can only increase in severity, your joints will continue to be stiff and uncomfortable. Similarly, if you are constantly criticizing the way you look, your lack of self-love will be reflected in your body. Your shoulders will slump and your countenance will be lackluster.

The first affirmation exercise gives you a series of statements to promote a sense of physical health and well-being. Using these affirmations may create a feeling of greater vigor and vitality by changing your negative beliefs about your body and health into positive ones. The second affirmation exercise helps to promote self-esteem and self-confidence. This is important in improving a low energy level. Many women with chronic fatigue lose their self-confidence and feel depressed and defeated by their condition. They feel frustrated and somehow at fault for not finding a solution. Use either or both exercises on a regular basis to promote healthful, positive thought patterns.

Exercise 7: Energizing Affirmations

- My body is strong and healthy.

- I have all the energy I need for healthy physical and emotional functioning.

- My endocrine glands are healthy; they function perfectly.

- My thyroid gland is healthy and makes just the right amount of hormones.

- My ovaries produce the levels of estrogen and progesterone that I need.

- My adrenal glands are healthy and can handle stress by producing the level of hormones that I need.

- My body chemistry is balanced and healthy.

- My immune system functions perfectly and protects me from infections and allergies.

- I handle stress and tension appropriately and effectively.

- My mood is calm and relaxed.

- I eat a well-balanced and nutritious diet.

- I enjoy eating delicious and healthful food.

- My body wants food that is easy to digest and high in vitamins and minerals.

- I do regular exercise in a relaxed and enjoyable manner.

- I practice the relaxation methods that I enjoy.

Exercise 8: Self-Esteem Affirmations

- I am filled with energy, vitality, and self-confidence.

- I am pleased with how I handle my health needs.

- I know exactly how to manage my daily schedule to accommodate my energy level.

- I listen to my body's needs and regulate my activity level to take care of my body's needs.

- I love and honor my body.

- I fill my mind with positive and self-nourishing thoughts.

- I am a wonderful and worthy person.

- I deserve health and vitality.

- I have total confidence in my ability to heal myself.

- I feel radiant with abundant energy and vitality.

- The world around me is full of radiant beauty and abundance.

- I am attracted only to those people and situations that support and nurture me.

- I appreciate the positive people and situations that are currently in my life.

- I love and honor myself.

- I enjoy my abundant energy and vitality.

Putting Your Stress-Reduction Program Together

This chapter has introduced many different ways to reset your mind and body to combat chronic fatigue. Try each exercise at least once. Experiment until you find the combination that works for you. Doing all eight takes no longer than 20 to 30 minutes, depending on how much time you wish to spend with each one. Ideally, you should do the exercises daily for at least a few minutes. Over time, they will help you gain insight into your negative beliefs and change them into positive new ones. Your ability to cope with stress should improve tremendously.

Suggested Reading

Benson, R., and M. Klipper. *Relaxation Response.* New York: Avon, 1976.

Brennan, B. A. *Hands of Light.* New York: Bantam, 1987.

Davis, M. M., M. Eshelman, and E. Eshelman. *The Relaxation and Stress Reduction Workbook.* Oakland, CA: New Harbinger Publications, 1982.

Gawain, S. *Creative Visualization.* San Rafael, CA: New World Publishing, 1978.

Gawain, S. *Living in the Light.* Mill Valley, CA: Whatever Publishing, 1986.

Kripalu Center for Holistic Health. *The Self-Health Guide.* Lenox, MA: Kripalu Publications, 1980.

Loehr, J., and J. Migdow. *Take a Deep Breath.* New York: Villard Books, 1986.

Miller, E. *Self-Imagery.* Berkeley, CA: Celestial Arts, 1986.

Ornstein, R., and D. Sobel. *Healthy Pleasures.* Reading, MA: Addison-Wesley, 1989.

Padis, E. *Your Emotions and Your Health.* Emmaus, PA: Rodale Press, 1986.

8

Breathing Exercises

*T*herapeutic breathing is of major benefit to women suffering from chronic fatigue; in fact, I strongly recommend its use in any chronic fatigue healing program. Women who are tired tend to restrict their movements in general. They exercise less, go out socially less frequently, and even restrict their household tasks. They spend more time lying on the bed or couch. When movement is limited in this way, breathing tends to become shallow and restricted. Instead of the deep abdominal breathing that we see with healthy aerobic activity, fatigued women may find that they practically stop breathing altogether and hold their breath for prolonged periods of time without even realizing it. The end result is a decrease in oxygen levels in the body, poorer blood circulation, muscle tension, and a decrease in metabolic activity of the cells.

Deep, slow abdominal breathing is essential for taking in large amounts of oxygen from the environment. Oxygen moves from the air you inhale, first into your lungs, and then into your circulation, where it binds to the red blood cells while traveling through the arteries and veins. Oxygen enables the cells to produce and utilize energy as well as remove waste products through the production of carbon dioxide, which you eliminate by exhaling. Your entire body needs optimal levels of oxygen for its normal cycle of building, repair, and elimination.

Therapeutic breathing exercises help enhance oxygenation and healthy body function. Try all the exercises in this chapter, then practice on a regular basis the ones you like the most. Pay attention to your breathing habits; if you catch yourself breathing shallowly or infrequently, correct this tendency by using the breathing techniques in this chapter. It is important to do the breathing exercises in a slow and regular manner. First, find a comfortable position. You'll do some exercises lying on your back, others sitting up. Unless otherwise directed, keep your arms and legs uncrossed and your back straight.

Exercise 1: Deep Abdominal Breathing

Abdominal breathing is a very important technique for the relief of chronic fatigue and for improving energy and vitality. Deep, slow breathing brings adequate oxygen, the fuel for metabolic activity, to all the tissues of your body. In contrast, rapid, shallow breathing decreases the oxygen supply and keeps you tired and devitalized. Deep breathing helps release tension and anxiety and relaxes the entire body. It also helps balance many other physiological processes such as pulse rate and hormonal output so that you can conserve and build your energy level, thereby healing chronic fatigue.

- Lie flat on your back with your knees pulled up. Keep your feet slightly apart. Try to breathe in and out through your nose.

- Inhale deeply. As you breathe in, allow your stomach to relax so that the air flows into your abdomen. Your stomach should balloon out as you breathe in. Visualize your lungs filling up with air so that your chest swells out.

- Imagine that the air you breathe is filling your body with energy.

- Exhale deeply. As you breathe out, let your stomach and chest collapse. Imagine the air being pushed out, first from your abdomen and then from your lungs.

- Repeat this exercise 10 times.

Exercise 2: Energy Breathing

This exercise combines imagery with deep breathing. As you visualize the energizing effects that breathing has on your body, you actually begin to lay down a mental blueprint for enhanced health and well-being. This exercise should leave you feeling peaceful with a greater degree of energy and ability.

- Lie flat on your back with your knees pulled up. Keep your feet slightly apart. Breathe in and out through your nose, if possible.

- Inhale deeply. As you breathe in, allow your stomach to relax so that the air flows into your abdomen. Let your stomach balloon out as you breathe in. Visualize the lowest parts of your lungs filling up with air.

- Imagine that the air you are breathing is filled with energy and vitality. See vitality filling every cell of your body. It fills you with a sensation of warmth and healing. Visualize this energy as a golden color. See the golden energy healing your body.

- Now, exhale deeply. As you breathe out, imagine the air being pushed out from the bottom of your lungs to the top.

- Repeat this sequence until your entire body feels relaxed and your breathing is slow and regular.

Exercise 3: Hara Breathing

In Oriental healing, the hara is one of the most important centers of vitality. In fact, it is called the "Sea of Energy." The hara point, located three finger-widths below the naval, is considered the center of the body in traditional Oriental healing models. Stimulation of the hara point helps to strengthen the body, as well as improve energy and endurance. Hara breathing nourishes and energizes the internal organs, improving health in general as well as decreasing chronic fatigue and tiredness.

- Sit upright in a chair, your arms at your sides. First, find the hara point with your fingers. Then, as you inhale deeply, draw breath into your lower abdomen and focus on concentrating your breath into the hara point. Feel the hara point expand and energize.

- As you exhale, see the hara point and your lower abdomen release the energy so that it circulates throughout your body.

- Repeat this exercise for several minutes—drawing breath and energy into the hara point as you inhale, then circulating energy throughout your body as you exhale.

Exercise 4: Breath of Fire

This short, rapid breathing technique is used in yoga to charge the body with immediate energy. This exercise also energizes the nervous system and stimulates blood circulation.

- Sit upright in a chair, your arms at your sides, palms up. As you inhale, fill your abdomen with a deep breath. Then breathe rapidly out through your nose, exhaling one short breath every second or two. As you breathe out, contract your abdomen by pumping in and out until your lungs are empty.

- Repeat several times until you feel energized and fully awake and present.

Exercise 5: Complete Body Breathing

This exercise promotes energy and vitality by directing your breath into every part of your body. This helps release stress and muscle tension in parts of your body that you aren't even aware are tense; it elevates the energy of the whole body. It reinforces the importance of the body functioning as a whole, integrated unit for optimal health and well-being. It also expands the electromagnetic field of the body through the use of color.

- Sit or lie in a comfortable position. Now, take a deep breath and visualize that the earth below you is filled with a bright cherry red color. This color goes 50 feet below you into the earth. Imagine that you are opening up energy centers on the bottoms of your feet. As you inhale, visualize the bright cherry red color filling up your feet. Draw this color up your legs and into your pelvic area and your lower back. As you exhale through your lungs, see this color flow out of your body and fill the air around you. Release any negative energy or emotions as you exhale, leaving the lower part of your body feeling clear and bright.

- Now inhale the bright red color up into your abdomen, chest, shoulders, and arms. See it filling your neck and head. As you exhale, see the bright red color flow out through your lungs and fill the air around you. As you breathe out, release any negative energy or thoughts and feelings until you feel bright and energized.

- Repeat this process 5 times.

Exercise 6: Glandular Breathing

Chronic fatigue often depletes endocrine gland function. Women with depleted endocrine glands may not only feel tired, but may also be prone to infections, because the endocrine glands help regulate immune function. Optimal endocrine function is very important for disease resistance, vitality, and energy. This exercise helps stimulate and energize your endocrine glands through the use of color breathing. When you direct your breath into the endocrine glands and visualize them being stimulated by the color, the glands receive better oxygenation and blood circulation. Nutrient flow to the glands is improved, as is the removal of waste products and toxins. The use of color expands the glands' electromagnetic energy field.

- Sit upright in a chair, your arms at your sides, palms up. Imagine that there is a large balloon filled with the color red above your head. This is a bright, vibrant tone of red that sparkles with energy. As you inhale deeply, see yourself popping this balloon and releasing the color red. See the color red flowing into your head and concentrating in the hypothalamus, a gland located at the base of the brain. As the hypothalamus begins to overflow with color, exhale and breathe the red out of your lungs, filling the air around you.

• As you inhale again, breathe the bright red color into your pituitary, an important endocrine gland located in your brain, right below the hypothalamus. Fill the pituitary with this color until it overflows. Then exhale deeply.

• As you continue to inhale the bright red color, let it flow into your thyroid gland, located in your neck, then into your thymus gland, located in the middle of your chest. Finally, let the color energize your adrenal glands, located in the middle of your back above the kidneys, and your ovaries, located in the pelvis. When you finish this exercise, relax for a few minutes.

Exercise 7: Muscle Relaxation Breathing

This exercise helps you get in touch with and release general muscle tension and tightness. Muscle tension is a common cause of chronic fatigue. By tensing your muscles, you cut off blood flow to vital organs and the brain and inhibit healthy muscle metabolism. When you are nervous and tense, or when you place your body in an awkward position while working or resting, you unconsciously tense up muscle groups throughout your entire body. The neck, shoulders, and back seem to be particularly vulnerable areas for stress, though other areas are prone to carry muscle tension, too. You can have tight and tense muscles in other parts of your body and not even be aware of it. This exercise helps focus on tension in your upper body. Relaxing and releasing the muscles in your neck and shoulders helps release muscle tension in your entire body. This is a good exercise to do while walking, playing sports, or doing desk work.

• Sit upright in a chair. Be sure you are in a comfortable position. Keep your feet slightly apart. Try to breathe in and out through your nose.

- Inhale and exhale deeply. As you breathe, let your head move from side to side. Keep your shoulders down and try to touch your ear to your shoulder. As you do this movement, imagine that your neck is made out of putty and that it allows your head to move in a supple, relaxed movement from the left to the right.

- Now inhale and pull your shoulders up toward your ears. Hold your breath and keep your shoulders in a hunched position. Exhale and let your shoulders drop back into a relaxed, comfortable position. Repeat this several times.

- Inhale and exhale deeply as you roll your shoulders forward. Make a large, slow, circular motion with your shoulders. Then, roll your shoulders back slowly. Repeat this several times.

- Inhale and exhale deeply, keeping the rest of your body still and relaxed. Repeat this several times.

Exercise 8: Emotional Healing Breath

I have seen, during my years of medical practice, that emotional stress is a significant trigger for chronic fatigue. This exercise uses breathing to help you release negative feelings such as chronic anger, hurt, or other upsets you may be harboring. The more time you spend cleansing old negative emotional patterns, the less impact these feelings will have on your energy levels.

- Lie flat on your back with your knees pulled up. Keep your feet slightly apart. Try to breathe in and out through your nose.

- Inhale deeply and see yourself enveloped in a soft white light. Breathe this light into every cell of your body. This is a cleansing light and can help wash away fear, anger, anxiety, and other negative feelings.

- As you exhale deeply, feel the light washing these emotions away.

- Repeat this exercise until you feel emotionally peaceful and clear.

Exercise 9: Depression Release Breathing

Depression often accompanies chronic fatigue. When a woman is tired, often her mood is low, too. It is hard to feel enthusiastic and high-spirited about life when you have no energy and vitality supporting your mental processes. This next exercise helps to elevate mood and enhance emotional wellbeing through focused breathing.

• Sit upright in a chair. Your arms are crossed in front of your chest with your fingers touching the upper outer area of your chest. Your wrist crosses over your heart chakra, which is the energy center for emotions and feelings in traditional Oriental healing models.

• As you inhale, imagine a golden light filling your heart center with a warm, loving feeling. As you exhale, breathe out depression and low spirits.

• As you inhale again, draw this golden light up through your neck and into your head. See it illuminating your head with a soft, peaceful glow. Feel any depression or negative thoughts dissolving as the golden light fills every cell in your brain.

• As you exhale, breathe the golden light out through the top of your head and see it form a shimmering cloud of energy around your entire body.

• Repeat the exercise 5 times.

Putting Your Breathing Exercise Program Together

This chapter suggests many effective exercises to help reduce fatigue through controlled breathing. Try each exercise once and choose those that you enjoy the most to practice on a regular basis. These exercises can help you even if you practice them only a few minutes each day. Over time, healthy breathing habits will become automatic and will greatly benefit your general health.

9

Light, Water,
& Sound

*T*his chapter describes several very useful and effective antistress techniques based on the therapeutic use of light, water (hydrotherapy), and sound. The techniques also affect your body's physiology and chemistry, benefiting your immune system as well as your endocrine or glandular system and promoting better circulation and muscle relaxation. Light, water, and sound therapy are delightful to use; you may find that they significantly improve the quality of your life.

Light Therapy

Many women with chronic fatigue feel worse during the winter months. Along with fatigue, they notice a deepening depression, weight gain, lowered body temperature, difficulty awakening in the morning, daytime drowsiness, and an increased craving for sweets. People affected with these symptoms tend to withdraw socially and experience a drop in their work performance. Researchers who have studied this problem over the past few decades call it Seasonal Affective Depression (or by its acronym, SAD); they have found that it is triggered by the decreased hours of daylight in winter. Interestingly, they also learned that the problem is worse in northern latitudes, where the level of light decreases even more in winter. The prevalence of SAD symptoms, not surprisingly, ranges from 1 to 2 percent in Florida to 10 percent in Alaska. Scientists believe that a deficiency of daylight causes depression by altering the rhythms of our daily biological processes, called circadian rhythms, and by delaying nightly secretions of melatonin, a hormone involved in the regulation of sleep. Those who suffer from SAD may also have disturbances in production of other chemicals that carry messages from one brain cell to another, such as dopamine and serotonin. Research studies suggest that vision also plays a role in causing SAD. Some women's eyes are less light sensitive and therefore less capable of taking in light efficiently during short winter days.

Women with SAD often spend more time indoors in winter, living and working under dim incandescent light or fluorescent lights, which lack the full range of outdoor sunlight. These women may greatly benefit from a daily one-hour walk in normal winter sunlight, since they will receive the aerobic benefits as well as the additional light exposure. Moreover, daily exposure to artificial bright light that simulates daylight for a week or two in the winter appears to be a powerful treatment for chronic fatigue and depression. More than 60 percent of people treated with this technique had dramatic relief of their symptoms. The therapeutic light exposure provides the best results if used in the early morning, but evening exposure also provides symptom relief. In either case, the individual experiences a greater total number of daylight hours. Currently, two treatment protocols are followed: (1) exposing an individual to a screen that emits light 5 times brighter than ordinary daylight for 2 hours each day, or (2) exposing an individual to a light panel that emits light 20 times brighter than normal room light for 30 minutes each day.

The LIFECYCLES Center has researched full spectrum light units and offers an excellent unit for individual purchase. See the Appendix for more information.

Hydrotherapy

Women with chronic fatigue may find a therapeutic bath extremely beneficial. It is a great way to unwind after a busy day or before going to sleep at night; many women find that a tub soak helps them sleep better. The warm water also loosens tight, constricted muscles and promotes better circulation to the muscles and skin. The healthy flush of the skin after a warm tub soak means the small blood vessels or capillaries have relaxed.

Hydrotherapy may take a number of different forms. Many women find bubble baths or bathing with scented floral oils relaxing as well as delightful to the senses. Some women set up the total bath environment to promote peace and relaxation by lighting candles, turning out the light, and soaking to classical music.

Women who own hot tubs or can use them at their local health club or YMCA have another powerful hydrotherapy tool for combating chronic fatigue. The combination of heat and water massage from the tub's small, powerful jets are very helpful in relaxing tight muscles and reducing tension. Hot tubs are particularly beneficial for women who suffer from insomnia, because heat appears to induce brain waves related to deep and restful sleep. Besides hydrotherapy, heat of any kind helps release muscle tension. You may want to try a hot water bottle or a heating pad to relieve muscle tension in particularly tight areas.

Following are two bath recipes I have found to be helpful for women with chronic fatigue.

Recipe 1: Alkaline Bath

This recipe is particularly good for women with chronic fatigue who need to relax tense, constricted muscles, as well as calm their anxiety and irritability. To a tub of warm water, add one cup of sea salt and one cup of bicarbonate of soda. I recommend using this highly alkaline mixture only once or twice a month. Soak for 20 minutes.

You will probably feel very relaxed and sleepy after this bath.

Use it at night before going to sleep. You will probably wake up feeling refreshed and energized.

Recipe 2: Hydrogen Peroxide Bath

This bath is energizing as well as useful in inducing muscle relaxation. Hydrogen peroxide is a combination of water and oxygen, so by adding it to your bath, you "hyperoxygenate" your water. The use of hydrogen peroxide improves the water quality, making the bath itself more pleasant. Hydrogen peroxide is quite inexpensive and can be purchased at any local drugstore and most supermarkets. I usually add three bottles of the 3 percent solution to a full tub of warm water and soak for up to half an hour. If you use the stronger peroxide (35 percent solution), add only 6 ounces to a full tub of water and avoid direct contact with your hands and eyes. Store this more concentrated peroxide in a cool place because it is a very powerful oxidizer.

Sound Therapy

Music can have a profound effect on both our moods and our physiology. Slow, quiet, classical music can help relax women whose chronic fatigue is worsened by constant upset, anxiety, and tension. Such music can slow pulse and heart rate, lower blood pressure, and decrease the output of stress hormones from the adrenal glands. When played before bedtime, it can help induce sleep for women suffering from insomnia. Tapes and records of nature sounds, such as ocean waves and rainfall, also have the ability to soothe and relax us. I have often used tapes of nature sounds in my home as a form of stress reduction for myself.

Music can also be a powerful healer for women whose chronic fatigue is accompanied by low spirits and depression. Certain kinds of music can act as a mood elevator, inspiring high spirits. Such music can improve energy and vitality and make us want to move, dance, and sing along. Many people find gospel and pop music particularly uplifting. Play music often to combat chronic fatigue, in your home, in your car, or as a background while you work.

Use the helpful suggestions in this chapter to set up your personal physical environment to combat chronic fatigue. These are some of my favorite techniques for increasing my own energy and vitality. By creating an environment that incorporates therapeutic use of light, water, and sound, you both improve your quality of life and reduce fatigue. These methods add grace and beauty to your surroundings, as well as promote healing. Try them all to see which approach helps you the most. For women living in a northern area of the country, light may be a significant factor in relieving fatigue, while sound and hydrotherapy may be more helpful for others. Find the combination that works best for you.

10

Physical
Exercise

$\mathcal{M}$any women with chronic fatigue simply stop exercising entirely because they lack the stamina and endurance to continue their habitual routines. I have seen in my practice many fit patients who were once regular joggers, bicyclists, or tennis players, but who stopped their activities altogether at the onset of chronic fatigue. Often these women became totally sedentary because their regular physical activities seemed to deplete their energy reserve.

This change from an active, athletic lifestyle to virtual inactivity is unnecessary for all but the most severe cases. Movement is the wellspring of life. Without the pulsation of the cells, the beating of the heart, and the contraction of the muscles, life ceases. Lack of exercise reduces circulation and oxygenation to vital organs, such as the brain and heart, and reduces the metabolism of all the cells of the body. On the other hand, women with chronic fatigue shouldn't be doing a prolonged, strenuous workout, since this will deplete the available oxygen and fuel supply of their muscles, making them feel more tired than ever. Thus, jogging, fast dancing, vigorous body building, and a hard game of tennis are not desirable activities for women with chronic fatigue.

An optimal exercise program for chronic fatigue includes slower, gentler activities that promote muscle and joint flexibility, reduce stiffness and muscle tension, and help increase good blood circulation and oxygenation to the entire body. The possibilities include walking, stretching, deep breathing exercises, range-of-motion and flexibility exercises, and gentle swimming to help keep a woman fit without stressing the body to the point of exhaustion. It is important to monitor your tolerance for exercise; women in the healing phase of chronic fatigue should never overdo any physical activity. For example, if you find that walking a mile makes you too tired, try walking half that distance. If your fatigue is really severe, then just deep breathing and flexibility exercises will be quite helpful if you are housebound for a period of time.

Exercise of any type helps keep a woman with chronic fatigue from feeling too depressed and blue. Many of my chronic fatigue patients complain of really low moods that hamper their quality of life and their effectiveness in solving the underlying health problems. Exercise helps oxygenate the brain and nervous system and promote healthy brain chemistry. By improving circulation, exercise facilitates proper nutrient flow and waste product removal. In fact, many of my patients find so much benefit in physical exercise as a way to reduce chronic fatigue and depression that it becomes their most effective form of stress management. They find that exercise produces a sense of peace and well-being unmatched by anything else they do.

This chapter provides a sequence of easy-to-follow exercises that you can use in your self-help program to improve your vitality and promote a sense of emotional well-being. You may want to combine them with gentle aerobic exercises such as walking. You can also combine them with yoga stretches (Chapter 11) and the use of acupressure massage (Chapter 12).

Guidelines for Physical Exercise

An exercise program for women with chronic fatigue, of necessity, must be gentle and not make too many demands on the body. Too strenuous an exercise program can leave a woman feeling more exhausted than ever. Therefore, I have included in this program only routines that promote blood flow and oxygenation to the vital organs as well as the muscles, decrease muscle stiffness and tension, and help loosen the joints. Since depression and chronic fatigue frequently co-exist, I have included mood-elevating exercises that can help you regain the zest for life that so many women with chronic fatigue feel is missing. You may also find these exercises helpful during times of increased emotional stress and tension.

Before you begin the exercise program for chronic fatigue, read through the following guidelines. These will allow you to perform the exercises in an optimal manner and without creating undue stress.

- Do all of these exercises during the first week or two of your program. Try each exercise at least once, then put together your own routine. You may find that you want to use all of them on a regular basis, or perhaps only a few. You can use any of these as warm-ups before participating in sports or athletic events.

- Perform the exercises in a relaxed and unhurried manner. Be sure to set aside adequate time—as much as 30 minutes—so that you don't feel rushed. Your exercise area should be quiet, peaceful, and uncluttered.

- Choose a flat area and work on a mat or a blanket. This will make you more comfortable while you do the exercises.

- Wear loose, comfortable clothing. It is better to exercise without socks to give your feet complete freedom of movement and to prevent slipping.

- Evacuate your bowels or bladder before you begin the exercises. Wait at last two hours after eating to exercise.

- Pay close attention to the initial instructions when beginning an exercise. Look at the placement of the body as shown in the photographs. This is very important, for you are much more likely to get relief from your symptoms if you practice the exercise properly.

- Try to visualize the exercise in your mind, then follow with proper placement of the body.

- Move slowly through the exercise. This will help promote flexibility of the muscles and prevent injury.

- Always rest for a few minutes after doing the exercises.

- Try to practice these movements on a regular basis. A short session every day is best. If that is not possible, then try to practice them every other day.

Exercise 1: Deep Breathing

Deep, slow abdominal breathing is essential for women with chronic fatigue. It expands your lungs and allows you to bring adequate oxygen, the fuel for metabolic activity, to all the tissues of your body. Rapid, shallow breathing decreases your oxygen supply and keeps you tired and devitalized. Deep breathing helps to relax the entire body and strengthens the muscles in the chest and abdomen. It helps to stabilize mood and reduce both depression and anxiety, so it is very important for emotional well-being.

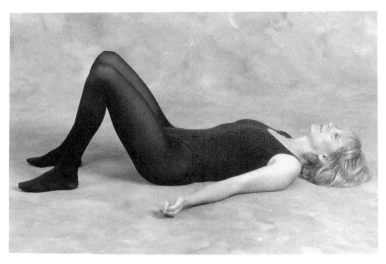

- Lie flat on your back with your knees pulled up or sit in a chair with your spine straight and your back supported. Keep your feet slightly apart. Breathe in through your nose and out through your mouth, making a "whoosh" sound.

- Inhale slowly and deeply. As you breathe in, allow your stomach to relax so that the air flows into your abdomen. Your stomach should balloon out as you breathe in. Visualize your lungs filling up with air all the way to the top so that your chest swells out.

- Imagine that the air you breathe is filling your body with energy.

- Exhale slowly and deeply through your mouth. As you breathe out, imagine the air being pushed out, first from your abdomen and then from your lungs. When all of the air is out, rest a few seconds and continue the breathing exercise.

Exercise 2: Total Body Muscle Relaxation

Women with chronic fatigue tend to have poor muscle tone. They frequently have muscle groups that are tense and tight because of inadequate oxygenation and blood flow. Lactic acid tends to accumulate in these muscles, and muscle tension can become a chronic problem. Regular physical activity effectively breaks up this pattern of chronically tight muscles. Unfortunately, women with chronic fatigue tend to become less active as their tiredness worsens. Although strenuous exercise is often too difficult for a woman with chronic fatigue, it is still very important to keep the muscles loose and flexible. Supple muscles have a beneficial effect on mood and induce a sense of peace and calm. The following exercise helps you to get in touch with the parts of your body that feel tense and contracted. It will also aid in releasing muscle tension.

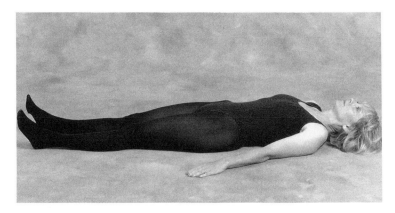

- Lie in a comfortable position. Allow your arms to rest limply, palms down, on the surface next to you. Practice your deep abdominal breathing as you do this exercise.

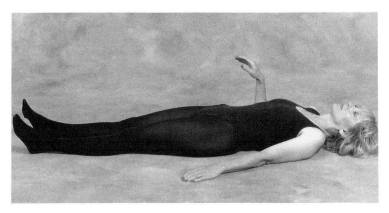

- Raise your right hand off the floor and hold it there for 15 seconds. Notice any tension in your forearm or upper arm. Let your hand slowly relax and rest on the floor. The hand and arm muscles should relax. As you lie there, notice any other parts of your body where you are carrying tension.

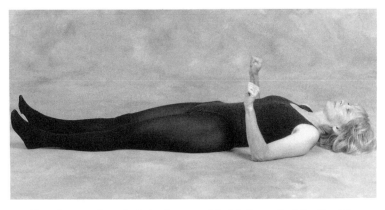

- Clench your hands into fists and hold them tightly for 15 seconds. As you do this, relax the rest of your body. Then let your hands relax.

- Now, tense and relax the following parts of your body in this order: face, shoulders, back, stomach, pelvis, legs, feet, and toes. Hold each part tensed for 15 seconds and then relax your body for 30 seconds before going on to the next part.

- Visualize the tense part contracting, becoming tighter and tighter. While relaxing, see the energy flowing into the entire body like a gentle wave, making all the muscles soft and pliable.

- Finish the exercise by shaking your hands. Imagine the remaining tension flowing out of your fingertips.

Exercise 3: Energizing Sequence

This exercise sequence is excellent for increasing your energy, releasing muscle tension, and improving circulation. Many women feel increased vitality and vigor upon completing this set. The exercise stimulates movement and energy flow through all muscles of the body, starting from the legs and moving up to the top of the head. In traditional Oriental healing models, these exercises are thought to stimulate the seven chakras or vital energy centers of the body.

Do the steps in this sequence slowly, to avoid stressing the body. You will better feel the benefits of this exercise if you don't rush through the steps or do them too hard. As your strength and flexibility improve, you may want to do the steps a little more vigorously.

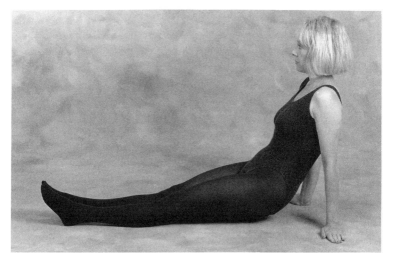

Legs and Hips

- Sit on the floor with your legs stretched straight in front of you. Place your hands on the floor behind you. Lift your buttocks off the floor and balance gently on the base of your spine.

- Repeat 5 times.

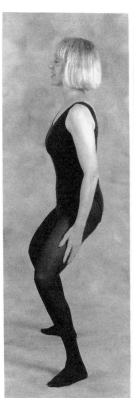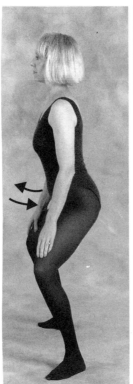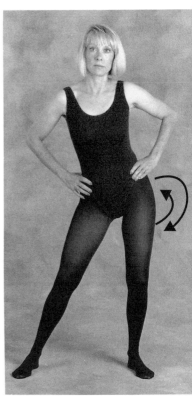

Legs and Pelvis

- Stand with your legs spread about 2 feet apart. Point your feet out at a comfortable angle.

- Rock your pelvis back and forth.

- Repeat 10 times. Then, rotate your hips in a circular fashion, first moving them clockwise and then counterclockwise.

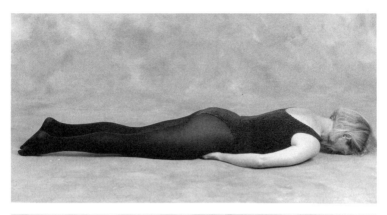

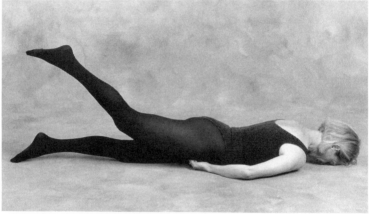

Pelvis and Lower Abdomen

- Lie on your stomach, placing your fists under your hips. Rest your forehead on the floor.

- As you inhale, raise your right leg with an upward thrust, keeping your hips on your fists. Hold for 5 to 20 seconds if possible.

- Lower the leg and slowly bring it back to the original position.

- Repeat several times. Then do the exercise on the left side.

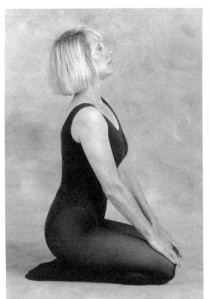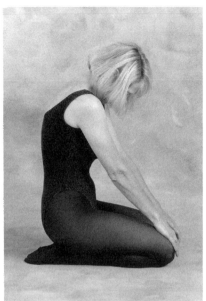

Abdomen and Chest

- Sit on your heels with your hands placed on your knees. As you inhale, arch your back and stretch your chest up and out in an expanded fashion.

- As you exhale, slump down to curve your back.

- Repeat several times.

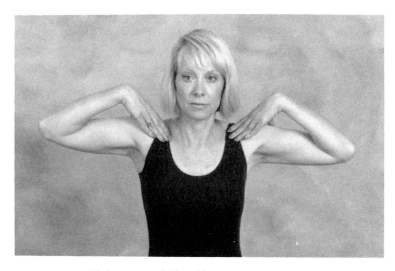

Abdomen and Shoulders

- Sit on the floor with your legs out in front. Raise your arms to shoulder level, bending them at the elbow.

- Place your hands on your shoulders with your fingers in front and thumbs in back.

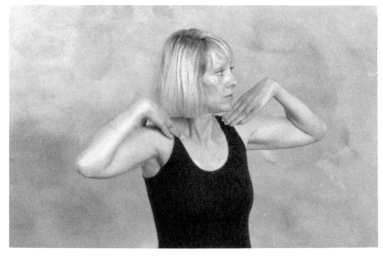

- Turn your elbows, head, and neck to the left and then to the right.

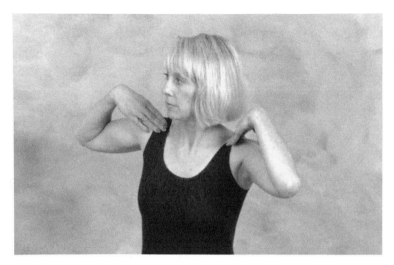

- Repeat 10 times. Be sure to let your entire torso move with your shoulders and arms.

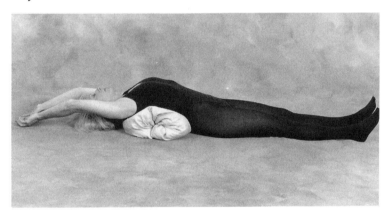

Back and Chest

- Lean backward over a hassock or a big soft pillow, so that your chest opens and expands as your shoulders go backward.

- Let the muscles of your chest relax.

- Keep your feet firmly on the floor.

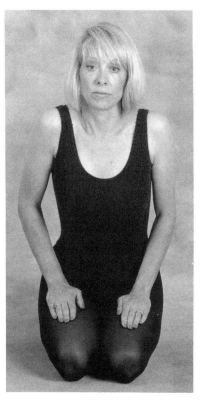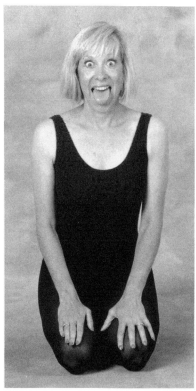

Neck

- Sit on your knees with your hands on your thighs. Take a deep breath and stretch your body upward.

- As you exhale, widen your eyes, stick out your tongue and push your body forward. Hold this position to the count of 10.

- Repeat this exercise 5 times.

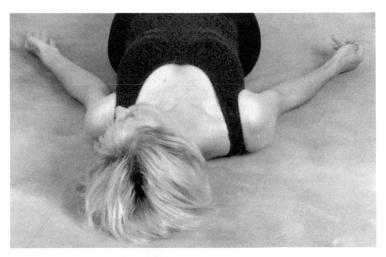

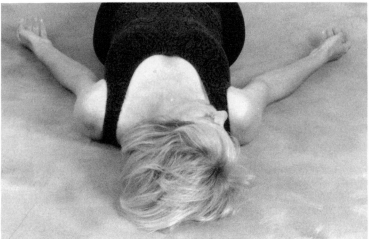

Neck

- Lie flat on your back on the floor in a relaxed manner.

- As you inhale, slowly turn your head to the left. Then, exhale as you return your head to the center position.

- As you inhale again, turn your head to the right. Continue this exercise for 1 minute.

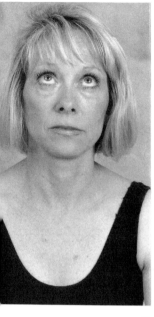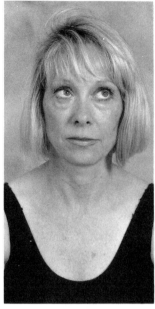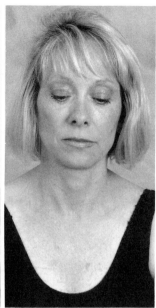

Eyes

- With your head facing straight and your facial muscles relaxed, roll your eye muscles in the following directions: up and down, and side to side.

- Move your eye muscles up to the left and down to the right.

- Reverse, moving your eyes up to the right and down to the left.

Head

- Lie on your back. Your arms should be at your sides, palms up.

- Close your eyes and relax your whole body.

- Inhale and exhale slowly, breathing from the diaphragm.

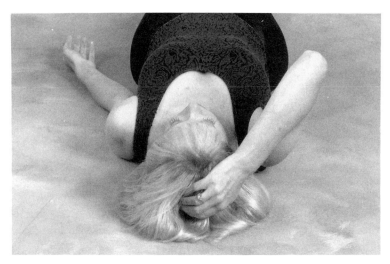

- Rub the crown of your head in a clockwise motion with your right hand for 30 seconds.

Activity Chart for Chronic Fatigue

Lower body exercise:	Walking
Upper body exercise:	Weight lifting (low impact)
Whole body exercise:	Swimming Ballroom dancing Golf
Flexibility exercise:	Yoga T'ai chi

Benefits of Exercise

- Improves oxygenation and blood circulation to the entire body.

- Improves functions of vital organs, including nervous system and digestive tract.

- Improves flexibility and decreases joint and muscle stiffness.

- Relieves depression, insomnia, anxiety, and irritability.
- Improves physical stamina and endurance.
- Increases your vigor and energy.

Suggested Reading

Caillet, R., M.D., and L. Gross. *The Rejuvenation Strategy*. New York: Pocket Books, 1987.

Hanna, T. *Somatics*. Reading, MA: Addison-Wesley, 1988.

Huang, C. A. *Tai Ji*. Berkeley, CA: Celestial Arts, 1989.

Jerome, J. *Staying Supple*. New York: Bantam Books, 1987.

Kripalu Center for Holistic Health. *The Self-Health Guide*. Lenox, MA: Kripalu Publications, 1980.

McLish, R., and V. Joyce, Ph.D. *Perfect Parts*. New York: Warner Books, 1987.

Pinkney, C. *Callanetics: 10 Years Younger in 10 Hours*. New York: Avon, 1984.

Solveborn, S. A., M.D. *The Book About Stretching*. New York: Japan Publications, 1985.

Tobias, M., and M. Stewart. *Stretch and Relax*. Tucson, AZ: The Body Press, 1985.

Yoga for Relief of Chronic Fatigue

*M*any different yoga stretches can improve your level of energy and vitality while you're healing from chronic fatigue. Practiced slowly and gently, these exercises can provide many physiological and emotional benefits for your body. A good yoga routine stretches every muscle in the body, promoting limberness and flexibility in the muscles and joints. At the same time, better circulation and oxygenation to the whole body stimulates metabolism and improves cell function. Improving circulation and nutrient flow to the brain and nervous system promotes healthy brain chemistry. This helps improve your mood, relieve depression, and reduce fatigue. Best of all, yoga is such an easy and gentle form of exercise that it can be practiced by most people, even women with severe chronic fatigue. Yoga is one of the few forms of physical activity that will not tire out a woman who has low physical reserve and stamina. When practiced on a regular basis, a good yoga routine can be an important part of your self-help program to regain your vigor and vitality.

When doing the exercises, it is important that you focus and concentrate on the positions. First your mind visualizes how the exercise is to look, and then your body follows with the correct placement of the pose. The exercises are done through slow, controlled stretching movements. This slowness enables you to have greater control over your body movements. You minimize the possibility of injury and maximize the benefit to the particular part of the body you are stretching. Follow the breathing instructions provided in the exercise. Most important, do not hold your breath. Allow your breath to flow in and out easily and effortlessly.

When beginning an exercise, pay close attention to the initial instructions. Look at the placement of the body as shown in the photographs. This is very important, because if you practice the pose properly, you are much more likely to get relief from your symptoms.

If you practice these yoga stretches regularly in a slow, unhurried fashion, you will gradually loosen your muscles, ligaments, and joints. You may be surprised at how supple you can become over time. If you experience any pain or discomfort, you have probably overreached your current ability and should immediately reduce the amount of the stretching until you can proceed without discomfort. Be careful, as muscular injuries can take quite a while to heal. If you do strain a muscle, immediately apply ice to the injured area for 10 minutes. Continue to use the ice pack two to three times a day for several days. If the pain persists, see your doctor.

Stretch 1: Ragdoll
This exercise helps relieve fatigue by releasing tension in the shoulder blades. Tension in the shoulders blocks blood flow and oxygenation to the head and neck area, making you feel mentally tired and sluggish.

• Stand easily with your legs apart. As you exhale, drop your head and body slowly forward.

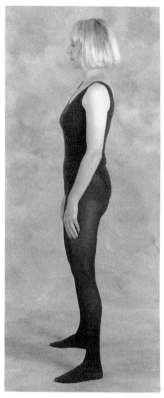
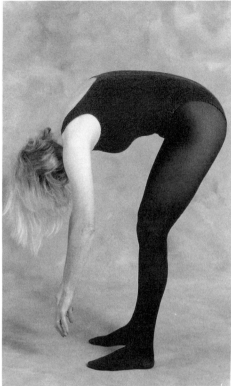

- Let your fingers hang down as close to the ground as possible. Deep breathe in this position for 30 seconds.

- Slowly come up to the standing position.

- Repeat 3 times.

Stretch 2: Chest Expander

This exercise increases circulation to the upper half of the body, energizing and stimulating the body. It also loosens and stretches tense muscles in the upper body, especially the shoulders and back, and expands the lungs.

- Stand easily. Arms should be at your sides; feet are hip distance apart.

- Extend your arms forward until your palms touch.

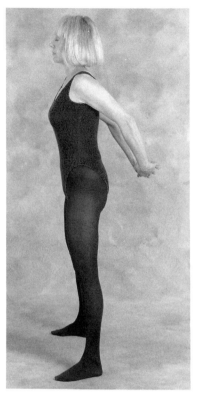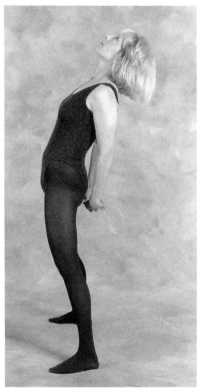

- Bring your arms back slowly and gracefully until you can clasp them behind your back.

- Exhale, then straighten your clasped hands and arms as far as you can without discomfort. Remember to stand upright; body should not bend forward. Breathe deeply into chest.

- Inhale deeply and bend backward from the waist. Keep your hands clasped and your arms held high.

- Drop your head backward a few inches and look upward as you relax your shoulders and the back of your neck.

- Hold this position for a few seconds.

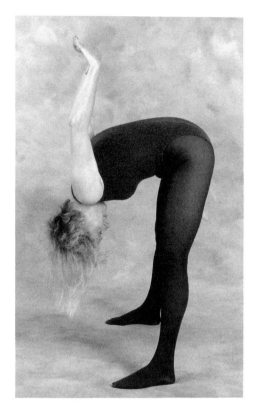

- As you hold your breath, bend forward at the waist, bringing your clasped hands and arms up over your back.

- Relax your neck muscles and keep your knees straight.

- Hold for a few seconds.

- Exhale as you return to the upright position. Unclasp your hands and allow your arms to rest easily at your sides.

- Repeat entire sequence 3 times.

Stretch 3: Rock and Roll

This exercise massages the entire neck, spine, and back muscles, as well as all the acupressure points along the spine. It will help to stimulate a sluggish thyroid by stretching and massaging the neck. This exercise will invigorate and energize you, reducing fatigue.

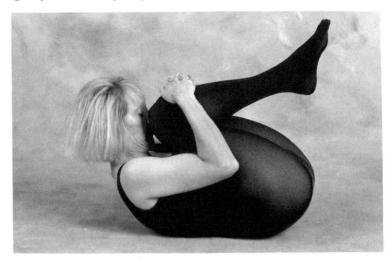

- Lie on your back. Bend and raise your knees to your chest, clasping them with your hands. Hands should be interlocked above knees.

- Raise your head toward your knees and gently rock back and forth on your curved spine. Note the roundness of your back and shoulders. Keep the chin tucked in as you roll back. Avoid rolling back too far on your neck.

- Rock back and forth 5 to 10 times.

Stretch 4: Boat Pose

This exercise helps to release overall body tension. It improves circulation and concentration. It helps to strengthen the lower back and abdominal area.

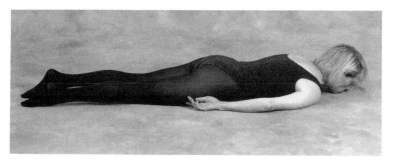

- Lie on your stomach with your feet together and your arms lying flat at your sides.

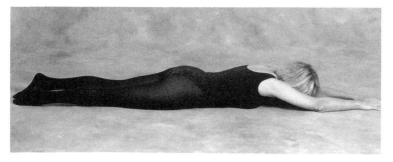

- Stretch your arms out straight in front of you on the floor.

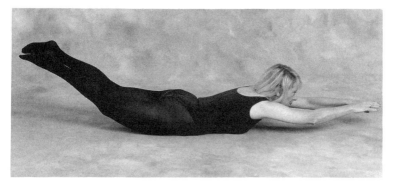

- As you inhale, arch your back and lift your arms, head, chest, and legs off the floor. Hold the pose as long as you can, up to 30 seconds, breathing deeply and slowly.

- Return to the original resting position with your head turned to the side, and completely relax for 1 to 3 minutes.

Stretch 5: The Locust

This exercise helps relieve PMS fatigue and other premenstrual and menopausal symptoms by energizing the female reproductive tract. It also energizes the liver, intestines, and kidneys. It strengthens the lower back, abdomen, buttocks, and legs.

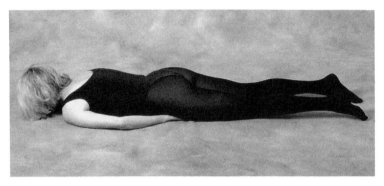

- Lie face down on the floor. Make fists with both your hands and place them under your hips. This prevents compression of the lumbar spine while doing the exercise.

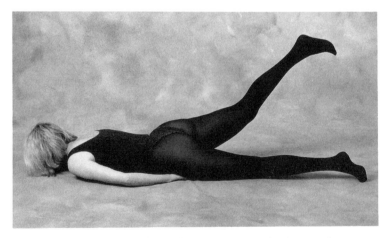

- Straighten your body and raise your right leg with an upward thrust as high as you can keeping your hips on your fists. Hold for 5 to 20 seconds if possible.

- Lower the leg and slowly return to your original position. Repeat with the left leg, then with both legs together. Remember to keep your hips resting on your fists.

- Repeat 10 times.

Stretch 6: The Bow

This exercise is one of the most powerful stretches for increasing total body energy and vitality and releasing muscle tension. It strengthens the nervous system, improves concentration and mental clarity, and relieves depression. It also stimulates the thyroid, thymus, liver, kidney, and female reproductive tract. It helps to improve digestive function and may reduce sugar craving.

- Lie face down on the floor, arms at your sides.

- Slowly bend your legs at the knees and bring your feet up toward your buttocks.

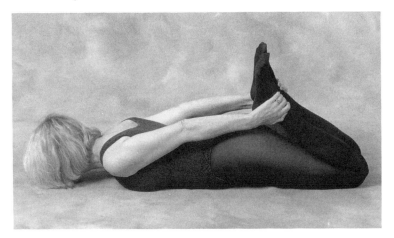

- Reach back with your arms and carefully take hold of first one foot and then the other. Flex your feet to make grasping them easier.

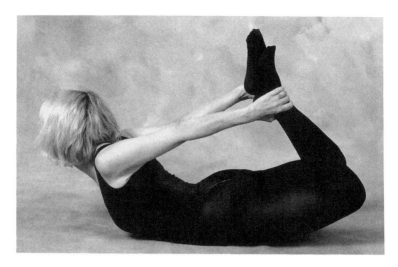

- As you inhale, lift your head and raise your trunk from the floor as far as possible. Bring your knees together and lift your legs off the floor as far as possible, too. Imagine your body looking like a gently curved bow. Hold for 10 to 15 seconds.

- Slowly release the posture. Allow your chin to touch the floor and finally release your feet and return them slowly to the floor. Return to your original position.

- Repeat 5 times.

Stretch 7: Half-Wheel Pose

This exercise improves your resistance to infections. Use it to help prevent colds and respiratory infections, to reduce the duration of a cold, or to relieve allergic and respiratory symptoms.

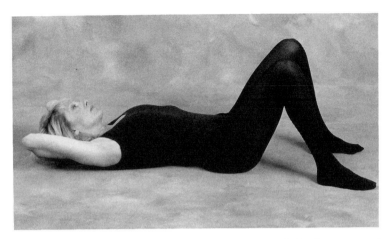

- Lie on your back with your knees bent and the bottoms of your feet flat on the floor.

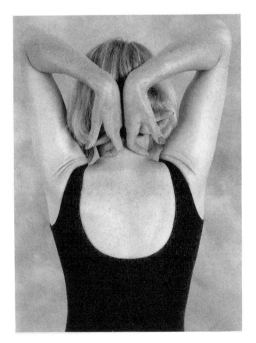

- Bring your hands under your neck with the backs of your hands pressing against each other and the knuckles of your smallest fingers pressing into the base of your skull. Spread your index finger and thumb apart on each hand.

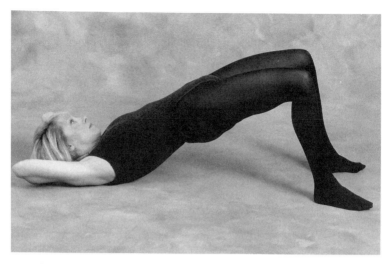

- Inhale deeply and arch your hips up. Breathe deeply in this position for up to 1 minute.

- As you exhale, slowly come down and return to your original position.

- Relax in this position for 1 to 3 minutes.

Stretch 8: Yoga Mudra

This exercise helps increase resistance to infections, particularly colds and flu, as well as decrease fatigue. It also helps clear tension around the shoulder blades.

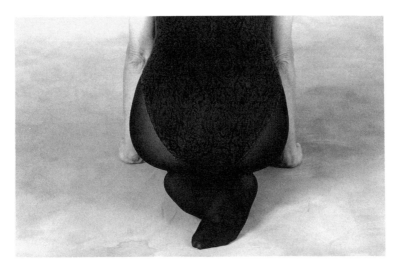

- Sit on your heels, placing the instep of one foot into the arch of the other.

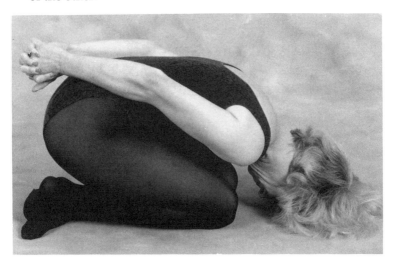

- Lower your head slowly forward to the ground, bringing your arms behind your back and interlocking your fingers. Be sure to have your palms facing each other.

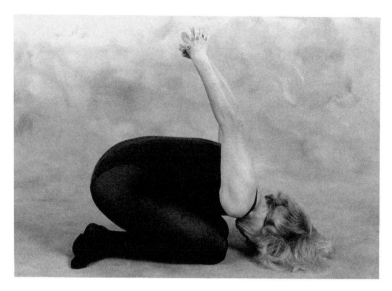

- As you inhale, raise your arms straight up, keeping your hands clasped together.

- Hold this position for up to 1 minute, breathing deeply.

- As you exhale, slowly unclasp your hands and let your arms relax on the floor, palms up.

- Relax in this position for 1 to 3 minutes.

Stretch 9: Side Rolls

This exercise helps relieve emotional tension and frustration. By helping release emotional upset locked in the muscles, side rolls promote a sense of relaxation, mental balance, and improved energy and vitality.

- Lie on your back with your hands interlaced under your neck.

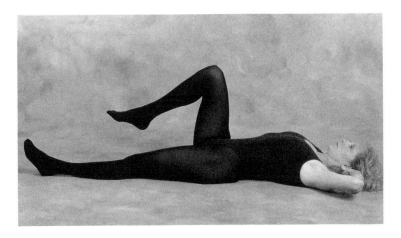

- As you inhale, bend and lift your right leg.

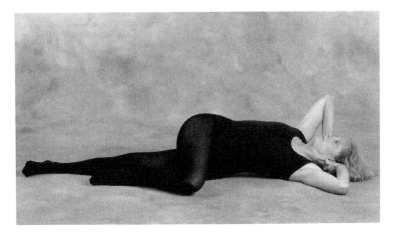

- Then exhale and roll on your left side, with your knee touching the ground. As you do this, release a sigh.

- As you inhale, return to your original position.

- Repeat this 10 times, alternating sides.

- Then relax on your back for 1 minute.

Suggested Reading

Bell, L., and E. Seyfer. *Gentle Yoga*. Berkeley, CA: Celestial Arts, 1987.

Couch, J., and N. Weaver. *Runner's World Yoga Book*. New York: Runner's World Books, 1979.

Folan, L. Lilias, *Yoga, and Your Life*. New York: Macmillan, 1981.

Iyengar, B. K. S. *Light on Yoga*. New York: Schocken Books, 1966.

Mittleman, R. *Yoga 28 Day Exercise Plan*. New York: Workman, 1969.

Moore, M., and M. Douglas. *Yoga*. Arcane, ME: Arcane Publications, 1967.

Singh, R. *Kundalini Yoga*. New York: White Lion Press, 1988.

Stearn, J. *Yoga, Youth and Reincarnation*. New York: Bantam, 1965.

12

Acupressure
for Relief of
Chronic Fatigue

*A*cupressure is an effective technique of Oriental massage that has traditionally been used to relieve chronic fatigue and improve energy, stamina, and endurance. Specific points on the skin are stimulated through gentle finger pressure that benefits energy levels. On the physical level, acupressure massage improves blood circulation, muscle tension, and other physiological functions.

On a more subtle level, acupressure is believed to release the body's supply of life energy to fight disease and promote healing. In Oriental medicine, this life energy is called chi; it is in some ways similar to electromagnetic energy. The chi is thought to run through the body in channels called *meridians*. When flowing freely, the chi moves through the meridians throughout the whole body, sometimes on the surface of the skin and sometimes deep inside the body, in the organs. Health occurs only when the chi is present in sufficient amounts and is equally distributed throughout the body, energizing all organ systems. When the energy flow in a meridian is stopped or blocked, disease occurs. Thus, acupressure massage is based on the belief that effective therapy restores and balances the body's energy. Stimulating the acupressure points on the skin surface corrects the meridian flow. When the normal flow of energy through the body is restored, the body is believed to heal itself spontaneously.

You can perform acupressure massage on yourself, or a friend can do it. Unlike acupuncture, acupressure does not require the use of needles, so it is safe, painless, and doesn't require years of specialized training. For years I have recommended that my patients use acupressure on specific points and have been very pleased with the results. Try the points mentioned in this chapter for relief of chronic fatigue and tiredness. You may find that acupressure massage is an important part of your personal self-help program.

Guidelines for Acupressure

Before you begin the acupressure exercises, read through the following guidelines. These guidelines will help you do the exercises correctly and make sure you receive the maximum benefit from them. I recommend that you try all the acupressure exercises during your first few treatment sessions. Then choose those that seem to benefit you the most and practice them on a regular basis.

- Try acupressure when you are relaxed. Make the room warm and quiet. Wash your hands and trim your nails to avoid bruising yourself. If your hands are cold, warm them in water.

- Work on the side of the body that has the most discomfort. If both sides are equally uncomfortable, choose whichever side you want. Working on one side seems to relieve the symptoms on both sides. Energy or information seems to transfer from one side to the other.

- Use the photographs that accompany the exercises to locate the points. Each point corresponds to a specific point on the acupressure meridians.

- Hold each point with a steady pressure for one to three minutes. Apply pressure slowly with the tips or balls of the fingers. It is best to place several fingers over the area of the point. If you feel resistance or tension in the area on which you are applying pressure, you may want to push a little harder. However, if your hand starts to feel tense or tired, lighten the pressure a bit. Make sure your hand is comfortable. The acupressure point may feel somewhat tender. This means that the energy pathway or meridian is blocked.

- Expect the tenderness in the point to go away slowly. You may also have a subjective feeling of energy radiating from this point into the body. Many patients describe this sensation as very pleasant. Don't worry if you don't feel it—not everyone does. The main goal is relief from your symptoms.

- Breathe gently while doing each exercise.

- Massage the points once a day or more, whenever you have symptoms of chronic fatigue.

Acupressure Exercises

Exercise 1: Use for Relief of Fatigue and Tiredness

This exercise helps relieve fatigue and tiredness. It stimulates the entire endocrine system because it involves a powerful point for the pituitary gland. This point also helps relax emotional tension as well as relieve eye strain, headaches, hay fever, ulcer pain, and indigestion.

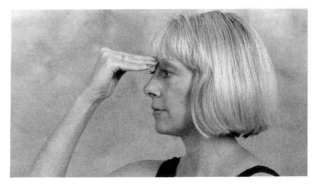

- Sit upright on a chair.

- Right hand holds point directly between the eyebrows, where the bridge of the nose meets the forehead.

- Hold the point for 1 to 3 minutes.

Exercise 2: Use for Relief of Fatigue, Depression, and Immune Dysfunction

This important sequence of points helps relieve upper body tension. The neck and shoulders generally carry a great deal of tension. Tightness in this area can act as a bottleneck and impede the energy flow of the entire body, thus releasing the tightness, energizing the entire body, and relieving fatigue. It also relieves depression and nervous tension. The points in this sequence also strengthen the immune system. A major treatment point for hypoglycemia is worked on in this exercise.

- Sit comfortably or lie down. Hold each step for 1 to 3 minutes.

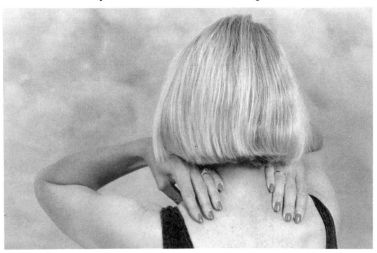

- Left hand holds point at the top of the left shoulder blade, 1 to 2 inches to the side of the spine. The point is between the shoulder blade and the spine. It may feel firm and resistant.

Right hand holds the same point on the right side.

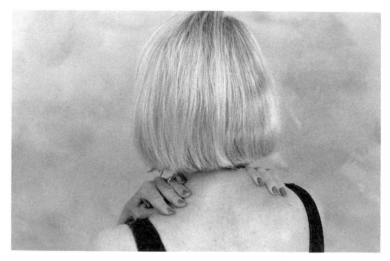

- Left hand holds point slightly to the back of the top of the left shoulder where the neck meets the left shoulder.

  Right hand holds the same point on the right side.

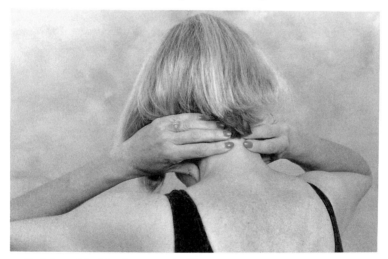

- Left hand holds the point halfway up the left side of the neck. Fingers sit on the muscle next to the spine.

  Right hand holds the same point on the right side.

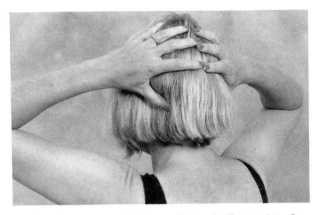

- Left hand holds the point at the base of the skull, 1 to 2 inches out from the spine.

Right hand holds the same point on the right side.

Exercise 3: Use for Relief of Fatigue and Tiredness

This exercise stimulates one of the most important acupressure points for energy, physical stamina, and power. The point stimulated in this exercise, termed the *hara* in Oriental medicine, is considered to be the body's center of gravity. This point also fortifies the digestive tract and helps to strengthen the reproductive system.

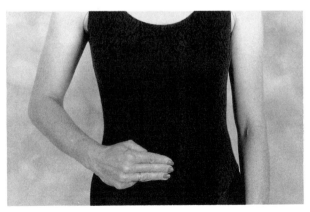

- Stand or sit upright on a chair.

- Fingers hold point below navel. Measure three finger-widths below navel to find this point. The point is located 1 to 2 inches deep inside the abdomen.

- Hold the point for 1 to 3 minutes.

Exercise 4: Use for Relief of Fatigue and Tiredness

This powerful energy point is one of the most important in Oriental medicine. It is used to quickly diminish fatigue and improve energy and endurance. Athletes have traditionally used it to tone and strengthen the muscles as well as increase stamina.

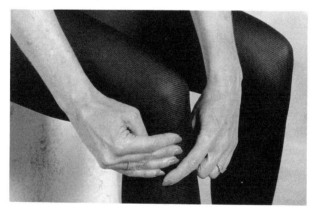

- Sit upright on a chair.

- Left hand holds point below right knee. This point is located four finger-widths below the kneecap toward the outside of the shinbone. It is sensitive to the touch in many people.

- Hold the point for 1 to 3 minutes.

Exercise 5: Improves Immune Function

This sequence of points strengthens the immune system and improves resistance to infections as well as relieving fatigue. This exercise also helps to prevent as well as relieve allergies. It balances the emotions and relieves symptoms of depression.

- Sit comfortably or lie down. Hold each step for 1 to 3 minutes.

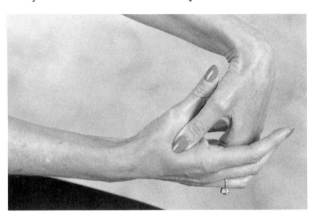

- Left hand holds point on right hand on the webbing between the index finger and thumb. Left thumb is placed on top of the webbing and the index finger is placed underneath the palm. The webbing is squeezed between the thumb and index finger.

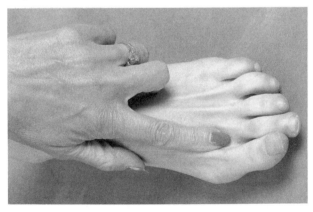

- Left hand rubs firmly the area between the bones at the top of the left foot below where the big toe and second toe meet.

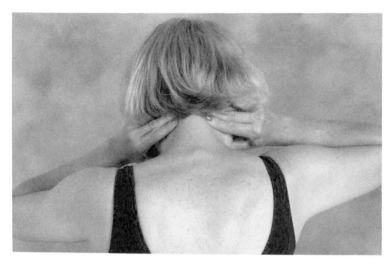

- Left and right hands hold points one-half inch below the base of the skull. Fingers will press on the ropy muscles on either side of the spine.

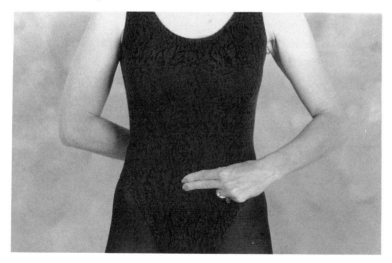

- Left hand holds point two finger-widths below the navel.

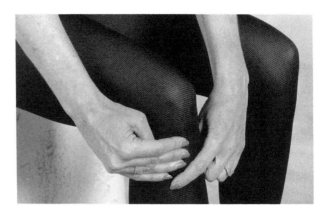

- Left hand holds point below right knee. This point is located four finger-widths below the kneecap toward the outside of the shinbone. It is sensitive to the touch in many people.

Exercise 6: Relieves Premenstrual and Menopausal Fatigue

This sequence of points relieves the fatigue that women experience prior to the onset of their menstrual periods. For many women with PMS, fatigue is a significant problem that recurs every month. This exercise can also help to relieve menstrual anxiety and depression, as well as menopause-related fatigue. The second step in this sequence has traditionally been forbidden for use by pregnant women after their first trimester.

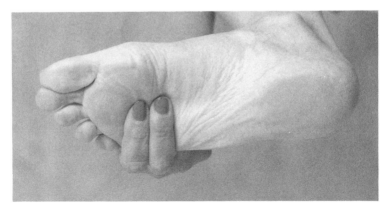

- Sit up and prop your back against a chair. Hold each step 1 to 3 minutes.

- Right hand holds point at the base of the ball of the right foot. This point is located between the two pads of the foot.

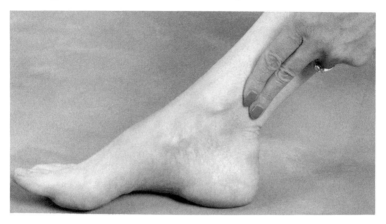

- Left hand holds the point midway between the inside of the right anklebone and the Achilles tendon. The Achilles tendon is located at the back of the ankle.

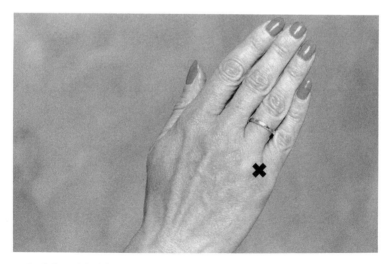

- Left hand holds point on right hand at the base of fourth finger.

- Repeat sequence on left side.

Exercise 7: Use for Relief of Thyroid Imbalance

This exercise energizes the thyroid, whose dysfunction can cause chronic fatigue and tiredness as well as excessive menstrual bleeding, anemia, constipation, and cold intolerance.

* Sit upright on a chair.

Hold each step for 1 to 3 minutes.

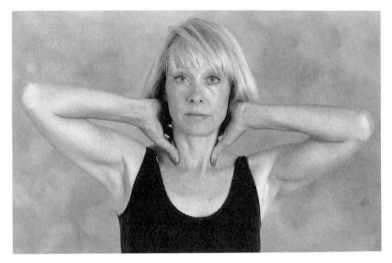

* Wrap hands around shoulders with thumbs pressing gently into both sides on top of collarbone.

* Fingers are in back. Press against upper shoulders and shoulder blade area.

Exercise 8: Use for Relief of Thyroid Imbalance

This exercise helps relieve chronic fatigue and tiredness due to thyroid imbalance. It is used to help stimulate the normal output of thyroid hormone.

* Sit upright on a chair.

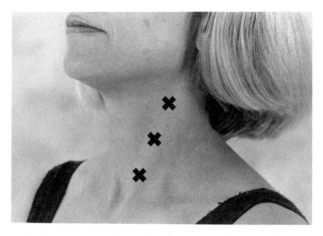

- Fingers touch three points along the large muscle on each side of the neck.

- Hold each point for 1 minute.

Exercise 9: Use for Relief of Anemia

This sequence of points is important for the treatment of anemia, a common cause of chronic fatigue and tiredness. It involves the stimulation of points on the spleen meridian, related to blood formation and menstrual problems.

- Sit upright on a chair. Hold each step for 1 to 3 minutes.

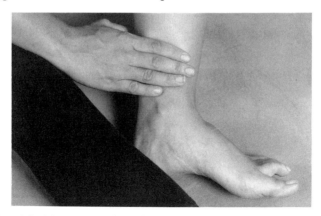

- Right hand holds a point four fingerwidths above the ankle bone.

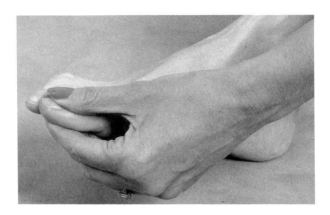

- Left hand holds a point over the big toe.

Suggested Reading

The Academy of Traditional Chinese Medicine. *An Outline of Chinese Acupuncture.* New York: Pergamon Press, 1975.

Bauer, C. *Acupressure for Women.* Freedom, CA: The Crossing Press, 1987.

Chang, S. T. *The Complete Book of Acupuncture.* Berkeley, CA: Celestial Arts, 1976.

Gach, M. R. *Acupressure's Potent Points.* New York: Bantam Books, 1990.

Gach, M. R. *Greater Energy at Your Fingertips.* Berkeley, CA: Celestial Arts, 1986.

Gach, M. R., and C. Marco. *Acu-Yoga.* Tokyo: Japan Publications, 1981.

Houston, F. M. *The Healing Benefits of Acupressure.* New Canaan, CT: Keats Publishing, 1974.

Kenyon, J. *Acupressure Techniques.* Rochester, VT: Healing Arts Press, 1980.

Nickel, D. J. *Acupressure for Athletes.* New York: Henry Holt, 1984.

Pendleton, B., and B. Mehling. *Relax With Self-Therap/Ease.* Englewood Cliffs, NJ: Prentice-Hall, 1984.

Teeguarden, I. *Acupressure Way of Health: Jin Shin Do.* Tokyo: Japan Publications, 1978.

13

Treating Chronic Fatigue with Drugs

$\mathcal{M}$ost cases of chronic fatigue do have treatable causes. It is important that all women with chronic fatigue have their symptoms evaluated medically by a physician so that any underlying causes can be treated with the appropriate medication. If your physician does prescribe medication, monitor its use carefully to avoid negative side effects. However, even in cases where medication may be important—such as hormonal replacement for low thyroid conditions or menopause—I find that combining the medication with self-help techniques gives the best results.

In this chapter, I describe the common drug therapies used for various causes of chronic fatigue. I focus particularly on treatments designed to alleviate fatigue symptoms. Ask your physician for more information about therapies that seem pertinent to your case.

Chronic Fatigue Syndrome

Drugs that block the production of stomach acid for the treatment of hiatus hernia, heartburn, and peptic ulcers have been used successfully to treat chronic fatigue patients. These drugs include such commonly used agents as Tagamet (cimetidine hydrochloride) and Zantac (ranitidine hydrochloride). Besides benefiting digestive function, these drugs also act as T-cell immune stimulants and block histamine receptors in T-cells. (Histamine is a chemical that can contribute to nasal congestion, itching, excessive stomach acid, and diarrhea.) These medications also improve energy, vitality, and alertness in women with CFS.

Doxepin is another histamine blocker that helps relieve CFS symptoms. It is a tricyclic antidepressant that may act as an immunomodulator. It has been used to relieve insomnia and induce deep, restful sleep in CFS sufferers. An added benefit for some people with CFS is the ability of doxepin to relieve muscle tension and tightness; it thus acts as a pain-relieving agent. Doxepin can also help relieve general fatigue, nasal congestion, gastritis, and neurological symptoms in CFS sufferers. Side effects include dry mouth, constipation, and weight gain. Other tricyclic antidepressants, such as Sinequan (doxepin hydrochloride) and Elavil (amitriptyline hydrochloride) are also used in CFS therapy.

Prozac (fluoxetine hydrochloride) is a relatively new antidepressant that may have immunomodulating properties. It acts by increasing the amount of serotonin available in the brain. (Serotonin is a neurotransmitter, a chemical that transmits messages from one part of the brain to another.) Prozac tends to help energize patients and relieve fatigue as well as other CFS symptoms. It does not improve sleep, however, and may actually worsen insomnia and anxiety in some women. Other side effects include rashes, digestive upsets, and impaired sexual functioning.

Gamma globulin provides passive immunity for people suffering from CFS through the injection of a blood product that contains antibodies. CFS sufferers tend to have low levels of IgG subclass I, which normally contains most of our antibodies effective against viruses. Gamma globulin therapy provides these particular antibodies, as well as a whole range of antibodies effective against many viruses, bacteria, and candida. It is also used for immunodeficiency disorders, such as the AIDS virus, leukemia, and lymphoma, and for autoimmune diseases such as idiopathic thrombocytopenic purpura, a bleeding disorder.

Gamma globulin is usually given in the intravenous form and is a very expensive form of treatment. CFS patients usually need two to three treatments per month, which can range from $500 to a $1000 per treatment. Side effects of this treatment include nausea, dizziness, transient flu-like symptoms, headache, and low blood pressure. Other biological drugs that may hold promise for CFS treatment by modulating the immune response include transfer factor, which triggers an active immune response, and alpha interferon, an immune enhancer.

Candida Infections

Physicians now commonly treat *Candida albicans* infections with three prescription medications. Nystatin, in use for 40 years, has been prescribed as an oral medication since the late 1970s to eradicate yeast in the intestinal tract. It is available in tablet, capsule, liquid solution, and powder form. Nystatin is used frequently to treat candida-infected patients who complain of fatigue, depression, headaches, and PMS symptoms. Nizoral (ketoconazole) is a newer antifungal medication that has been used in the United States since 1981. Nizoral has been used successfully by physicians for yeast infections that are more difficult to eradicate, along with a sugar-free diet (which should be used by all candida-infected patients). The medication may occasionally cause serious side effects. Because of this, liver function should be monitored every few weeks in women taking the medication for one month or more. Diflucan (fluconazole) is a broad-spectrum antifungal agent related to Nizoral. It is the most recently introduced of the three medications in the United States, although it has had previous use in Europe. Studies suggest that it is a more powerful antifungal agent than Nizoral and causes less toxic side effects.

Allergies

Antihistamine and decongestant medications are frequently used to control the common symptoms of allergy. Yet one of the main side effects of these medications is sedation. In fact, some women use antihistamines specifically for their side effects—to induce sleep—as an alternative to stronger sleep medication. Therefore, these drugs should be used cautiously by women with chronic fatigue, particularly in a work setting or when they are driving. A better approach is the eradication of allergens through an antifatigue, low-stress diet and the elimination of allergens from the physical environment, in order to reduce the dependence on antihistamines and decongestants in an allergic woman with chronic fatigue.

PMS and Depression

Depression caused by emotional factors, as well as PMS-related depression and fatigue, may be relieved by antidepressants. Antidepressant medications may help to correct the chemical basis of the underlying depression and often bring positive relief of symptoms within three to eight weeks. These medications should be used cautiously and only if the more gentle self-help treatments fail, because they are very powerful drugs and unfortunately can cause significant side effects. They should be used only when prescribed and supervised by a knowledgeable physician.

The most common antidepressant drugs prescribed have been the tricyclics such as Elavil and Tofranil (imipramine hydrochloride). They are particularly useful for depression accompanied by insomnia and weight loss. Tricyclics can cause sedation as a side effect, so women with chronic fatigue need to be alerted to this fact. Monoamine oxidase inhibitors such as Nardil (phenelzine sulfate) and Marplan (isocarboxazid) are used to treat depression involving phobias, sleeping too much, and weight gain. They are prescribed less frequently, because of their side effects. Prozac, a relatively new antidepressant, is being prescribed with increased frequency by physicians. Though it is quite effective in relieving depression, 12 percent of users report drowsiness as a side effect, a real problem for women with chronic fatigue. As with the other antidepressants, Prozac has other numerous side effects in susceptible users.

Women with PMS-related fatigue and depression need to be careful using some commonly prescribed PMS medications. Diuretics can be helpful in the short term for reducing PMS-related fluid retention and bloating. However, they also deplete the body's store of essential minerals, such as potassium and calcium. Over time, depletion of minerals can worsen chronic fatigue. England has pioneered the use of natural progesterone as a treatment for PMS, and some physicians in the United States prescribe it as a suppository or an oral tablet. Though progesterone can be a helpful treatment for PMS anxiety, irritability, and mood swings, women with PMS-related fatigue and depression should use it cautiously. Progesterone has sedative properties, and in high levels can be used as an anesthetic. If you have specific questions about the appropriateness of progesterone for treatment of your PMS, ask your physician. Some doctors occasionally prescribe birth control pills for PMS in an attempt to reduce symptoms by suppressing ovulation. The progestins or synthetic progesterone in oral contraceptives can worsen fatigue and depression, particularly if the pill is progesterone-dominant.

Menopause

Many menopausal women find that the use of hormonal replacement therapy gives their moods and energy levels a tremendous boost. With the use of estrogen and progestins (a synthetic form of progesterone) many of my patients have reported not only relief from hot flashes and vaginal dryness, but also more energy, mood stabilization, and improved sex drive. Depression, the blues, and fatigue are often eradicated, as are insomnia, irritability, and edginess.

Estrogen can be taken either in pill form or as a vaginal cream. There are many brands on the market, generally composed of combinations of two types of estrogen that occur naturally in your body: estrone and estradiol. Estrone is the main type of estrogen that your body makes after menopause, while estradiol is present in greater amounts during your menstrual years.

Both synthetic and naturally derived estrogen are available. The most popular brand is Premarin (conjugated estrogen tablets), which comes from the urine of pregnant mares and contains a natural mixture of estrogen, including estrone. Other popular brands include Ogen (estropipate tablets), which contains estrone; Estrace (estradiol tablets), which contains estradiol; and many other generic formulations.

When estrogen is taken as a pill, it is usually administered daily from the first to the twenty-fifth day of the month. About a week after taking the last pill, bleeding similar to a menstrual period will occur unless, of course, a woman has had a hysterectomy. A progestin (synthetic progesteronelike compound) is usually added for 10 days at the end of each 25-day course of estrogen because it seems to protect women from developing uterine cancer. For that reason, most doctors today prescribe a combination of estrogen and progestin for menopause symptoms. Common brands of progestins on the market include Provera (medroxyprogesterone acetate), Amen (medroxyprogesterone acetate), and Norlutin (norethindrone tablets).

Because of the possible side effects of using hormones, most physicians prescribe the lowest effective dose of both estrogen and progestins that relieves the patient's symptoms. Much higher doses were used several decades ago, both in estrogen replacement therapy and in birth control pills, but the current trend is definitely toward smaller doses of hormones to achieve the same beneficial effects. Women with a history of uterine or breast cancer, active fibroid tumors, endometriosis, liver or gall bladder disease, and vascular problems should avoid hormonal replacement therapy. Unfortunately, progestins like Provera can worsen fatigue and depression in susceptible women. Women with preexisting chronic fatigue should use them cautiously.

Occasionally, women in menopause may have to resort to the use of antidepressants if their fatigue and depression are not relieved by the use of hormones. Refer to the section on PMS medication for more specific information on common antidepressant medications.

Anemia and Hypothyroidism

In some cases drug therapy can correct anemia, if it addresses the underlying cause of the problem. For instance, hormonal therapy can help correct anemia caused by heavy menstrual bleeding. This problem is often seen in teenagers and in women who are in transition into menopause. The anemia may become particularly acute in premenopausal women because of hormonal instability. As their follicles lose the ability to produce estrogen and progesterone, premenopausal women begin to ovulate less frequently. The menstrual cycle often shortens, with periods coming closer together. Bleeding may become heavier and last longer. A menstrual period lasting 7 to 10 days is fairly common. In extreme cases, women may bleed 60 or more consecutive days. As menopause approaches, this instability corrects itself. Periods become farther apart, and the flow becomes lighter until menstruation finally ceases.

It is during the phase of heavy menstrual bleeding that women are most likely to need medical care. Often the bleeding can be stopped by a synthetic progesteronelike hormone called a progestin. Provera is the type used most often in the United States; administered orally for one or two weeks, this drug can usually stop the bleeding. It acts much the way natural progesterone does, by limiting the amount of bleeding from the uterine lining during the second half of the menstrual cycle. Although Provera can be quite effective in stopping heavy menstrual bleeding, it does cause side effects in some women; unfortunately, the most common is depression and fatigue. Therefore, Provera can act as a double-edged sword: correcting fatigue by stopping heavy bleeding and anemia, while worsening fatigue in some women.

Another treatable cause of anemia-related fatigue is low thyroid function. Hypothyroidism is easily treatable by thyroid replacement therapy. Besides correcting fatigue and tiredness, thyroid replacement therapy corrects other common symptoms of thyroid deficiency, including constipation, skin and hair changes, weight gain, excessive menstrual bleeding, and elevated blood cholesterol levels. A thyroid imbalance must be carefully managed by a physician through blood tests and office evaluation so the proper dose can be prescribed. Most people who suffer from thyroid conditions are female (90 percent of the total hypothyroid cases in the United States are women), so it is a common condition frequently seen by physicians who specialize in women's health care.

In conclusion, many drug therapies may be helpful in treating either the causes or symptoms of various forms of chronic fatigue. Unfortunately, quite a few of these drugs may have side effects that are quite difficult for women with chronic fatigue to handle. Check with your own physician for specific guidelines on these medications.

14

How to Put Your Program Together

*C*hronic *Fatigue & Tiredness* has given you a complete self-help program to help prevent and relieve your symptoms. The treatment chart on page 46 summarizes the many treatment options presented in this book. Refer to this chart as you put your personal program together. Try the treatment options that feel most comfortable to you. You may find that certain exercises or stress-reduction routines feel better to you than others. If so, practice the ones that bring the greatest sense of relief for your particular symptoms.

Don't get bogged down in details. Always keep in mind that your ultimate goal is relief of your chronic fatigue and a general improvement in your overall health and well-being. I usually recommend beginning any self-help program slowly so you can get used to the lifestyle changes comfortably. People differ in their ability to adjust to major lifestyle changes. Though some of my patients like to eliminate their old, unhealthy habits as quickly as possible, many other women find such rapid changes in their long-term habits to be too stressful. Find the pace that works for you.

Enjoy the program. I always tell my patients to regard their self-help program as an enjoyable adventure. The exercise and stress-reduction programs should give you a sense of energy and well-being. The menus and food selections I've recommended in this book provide you with an opportunity to try delicious and healthful new foods. As you do the program, don't set up unrealistic or overly strict expectations for yourself. You don't have to be perfect to get great results. Just follow the guidelines of the program as best you can and as your schedule permits.

It is not a disaster if you forget to take your vitamins occasionally or don't have time to exercise on a particular day. Don't be discouraged if you can't follow the dietary recommendations on vacations, holidays, and birthdays. Periodically review the guidelines outlined in this book and continue to adapt your lifestyle to the healthful suggestions that I've shared with you from my years of medical practice. Over time you will notice many beneficial changes.

Be your own feedback system. Your body will tell you if you are on the right track and if what you are doing is making you feel better. It will also tell you if your current diet and emotional stresses are worsening your symptoms. Remember that even moderate changes in your habits can make significant differences.

The Chronic Fatigue Workbook

Fill out the workbook section of this book. The workbook questionnaires will help you determine which areas in your life have contributed the most to your symptoms and need the most improvement. Review the workbook every month or two as you follow the self-help program. The workbook will help you see the areas in which you are making the most progress, with both symptom relief and the initiation of healthier lifestyle habits. The workbook can give you feedback in an organized and easy-to-use manner.

Diet and Nutritional Supplements

I recommend that you make all nutritional changes gradually. Many women find breakfast the easiest meal to change because it is simple and often eaten at home. To change your other meals and snacks, periodically review the lists of foods to eliminate and foods to emphasize provided in this book. Each month, pick a few foods that you are willing to eliminate from your diet. Try in their place the foods that help prevent and relieve chronic fatigue. The recipes and menus in Chapter 5 should be very helpful; use the meal plans as helpful guidelines while you restructure your diet to suit your needs.

Vitamins, minerals, essential fatty acids, and herbal supplements can help to complete your nutritional needs and speed up the healing process. Most women find these a very important part of their self-help program.

Stress Reduction and Breathing Exercises

The stress-reduction and breathing exercises play an important role in facilitating the physical healing process. I also suggest trying the light, water, and sound therapies for added relaxation. I find that all my patients heal more rapidly when they are calm, happy, and relaxed. The visualization exercises can help you set a blueprint in your mind for optimal health; this enables your body and mind to work together in harmony.

Begin the program by putting aside 15 to 30 minutes each day, depending on the flexibility of your schedule. Try all the stress-reduction and breathing exercises listed in this book. Choose the combination that works best for you. Practice stress management on a regular basis and be aware of your habitual breathing patterns. Both of these techniques will help you relax and release the tensions that worsen your fatigue. They will help induce a sense of peace and well-being.

You do not need to spend enormous amounts of time on these exercises. Even 10 minutes out of your daily schedule can be helpful. You may find that the quietest times for you are early in the morning before you get out of bed, or late at night before going to sleep. Or, you might choose to take a break during the day. You can close the door to your office or go into your bedroom at home for 10 minutes to relax. Use the time to breathe deeply, do the visualizations, or meditate. You will be much calmer and more relaxed afterward.

Physical Exercise

Women with chronic fatigue should do moderate exercise on a regular basis, at least three times a week. Aerobic exercise can help improve circulation and oxygenation, thereby helping you to relax. It is important, however, to do your exercise routine in a slow, comfortable manner, so as not to worsen your symptoms. Frenetic exercise that is too fast-paced is unhealthy if you are already fatigued; it can actually exhaust you further. Pick a tempo that feels relaxing and comfortable.

To do the yoga stretches and acupressure massage described in this book, I recommend that you set aside a half-hour each day for the first week or two of starting your self-help program. Try all the exercises. After an initial period of exploration, choose the ones that you enjoy the most and that seem to give you the most relief. Practice them on a regular basis so that they can help prevent and reduce your symptoms.

Conclusion

I wish to reaffirm that each of us can do a tremendous amount for ourselves to assure optimal health and well-being. By having access to information, education, and health resources, every woman can play a major role in creating her own state of good health. Practice the beneficial self-help techniques that I've outlined in this book. Follow good nutritional habits, exercise, and practice regular stress-reduction techniques.

By combining good principles of self-care along with your regular medical care, you can enjoy the same wonderful results that my patients and I have had for a life of good health and well-being.

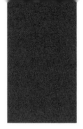

Appendix

Health and Lifestyle Resources for Women

The LIFECYCLES Center

*F*or many years, I have been a very strong advocate of the need for health and lifestyle resources that provide women with the information, education, and resources they need for optimal health and well-being. The more access that women have to information about their important health issues, the more they can participate in and promote their own well-being. I have worked with many thousands of women of all ages, both as patients and in classes I have given. I have been impressed by the intense desire that women have for information on how to stay healthy.

Unfortunately, finding information on major health issues has been difficult for most women. First of all, research on women's health issues has traditionally been a very low priority in the medical and scientific community. Few government dollars have been spent researching the major female health problems. In addition, any woman who is faced with the need to handle any significant female-related problem finds that there is an almost total lack of available information. Very little in-depth information is available on what women can do on their own to maintain their health and well-being. I get calls and letters from women all over the world looking for self-care resources for a variety of health issues. The necessary resources for women who want to practice good preventive health care are available through *The LifeCycles Center.*

The Center provides complete self-help programs and resources that address a variety of women's health care and lifestyle issues, including PMS, menstrual cramps, menopause, anemia, heavy menstrual bleeding, chronic fatigue and tiredness, and back discomfort. We will be adding a number of additional self-help programs in 1993. Self-help books on breast cysts and tumors, depression, fibroids, endometriosis, addictions, and migraine headaches will be available soon. I have spent the past 20 years gathering these resources and information. I use these techniques and products constantly in my own wellness program and recommend them for use by my patients. We currently stock the following resources for women:

Books by Susan M. Lark, M.D.

PMS Self-Help Book
Menopause Self-Help Book
Anemia and Heavy Menstrual Flow—A Self-Help Program
Menstrual Cramps—A Self-Help Program
Chronic Fatigue and Tiredness—A Self-Help Program
Fibroid Tumors & Endometriosis—A Self-Help Program
Anxiety & Stress—A Self-Help Program
Estrogen: Facts & Alternative Therapies

Foods

Flax Oil. Flax oil is the best food source of the essential fatty acids that are so important for women's optimal reproductive health. This oil has a delicious buttery flavor! Flax oil is delicate and should not be used for cooking, but adds great buttery flavor to popcorn, potatoes, rice, steamed vegetables, pasta, hot cereals, and many other dishes. Add to your food just before serving.

Flax and Borage Oil Capsules. This is a great way to take essential fatty acids as a supplement. I recommend that women take at least four capsules a day for nutritional support for dry skin and vaginal tissues, PMS cramps, and menopausal symptoms. Fatty acids are found throughout the body and provide important support to maintain optimal health and wellness in many body systems.

Flax Seed Powder. This makes a delicious cereal base. Just stir in apple juice or milk for a great tasting cereal. You can also sprinkle flax seed powder on cereals, casseroles, and desserts for a delicious nutty flavor.

Nondairy Milk. Vegelicious, a new potato-based milk, is absolutely fantastic. It contains 240 milligrams of calcium per 8-ounce serving. I strongly recommend its use for women with any type of menstrual problem, including PMS, menstrual cramps, and menopause. It is an excellent replacement for cow's milk since it does not contain the chemicals that worsen these common female conditions. It is also a great cow's milk substitute for adults and children with allergies and food sensitivities since it is easy to digest. Children love its taste. Use it as you would cow's milk.

Vitamin and Mineral Supplements Formulated Specifically for Women

These formulas have been developed by Susan M. Lark, M.D., and provide complete nutritional support for women who want to practice lifestyle and nutritional habits as part of their treatment programs for a variety of common female complaints.

PMS Nutritional System
Menopause Nutritional System
Woman's Daily Spectrum Nutritional System
Women's Daily Iron Nutritional System
Women's Water Balance
"Unwind," A Daily Relaxant
Bioflavonoids

Herbal Tinctures for Women

These herbs supply beneficial nutritional support for women. For chronic fatigue, combine these herbs according to the formulas in Chapter 6. The Center has them available in large 4- and 8-ounce sizes. Tinctures are the most economical and cost effective way to purchase herbs.

Yellow dock	Huckleberry
Oregon grape root	Turmeric
Wild yam	Shepherd's purse
Goldenseal	Sarsaparilla
Parsley	Black cohosh
Ginger root	White willow bark
Red raspberry leaf	Cramp bark
Chamomile	Hops
Chaste tree berry (Vitex)	Ginkgo biloba
Buchu	

Recipe Cards and Meal Plans

These recipe cards and meal plans have been developed by Susan M. Lark, M.D., based on her two decades of work in the field of women's health care and preventive medicine. Each packet provides women with delicious, easy-to-prepare meals that contain therapeutic levels of the nutrients that women need for good health.

Recipe Cards for Healthy Women—Breakfast
Recipe Cards for Healthy Women—Lunch and Dinner
Recipe Cards for Healthy Women—Snacks and Desserts

Women's Personal Products

Vitamin E Vaginal Suppositories. These suppositories help soothe the vaginal tissues.

Products for Muscle Tension, Back Discomfort and Stress Reduction

The Archable Body Bridge. This healthful device stretches the body naturally along its arc. It is a terrific tool to help increase overall flexibility, correct poor body alignment, and improve posture. Use it every day for relaxation and relief of muscle tension. This is a very useful device for women who tend to get menstrual cramps, because it stretches and relaxes tense pelvic and abdominal muscles. It can be particularly helpful for women who do sit-down work for long periods of time when they have menstrual cramps.

Full Spectrum Light Unit. The use of special full spectrum light units has been found to be very effective for the relief of seasonally related chronic fatigue and depression. *The LIFECYCLES Center* has an excellent unit available for women who are sensitive to seasonal changes.

The Voyager. This wonderful device uses sound and light to help guide women into a state of deep relaxation, sound sleep, and reduction of muscle tension.

Please contact the Center directly if you are interested in obtaining any of our self-help programs and resources for women.

The LIFECYCLES Center
101 First Street, Suite 441
Los Altos, CA 94022-2706
(415) 964-7268 (For information)
(800) 862-9876 (For orders only)

About Susan M. Lark, M.D.

Susan M. Lark, M.D., is a noted authority on women's health care and preventive medicine. She is Director of *The* LIFECYCLES *Center*. She also sees patients in her private practice in Los Altos, California. Dr. Lark has been on the clinical faculty of Stanford University Medical School, Department of Family and Preventive Medicine. Dr. Lark lectures widely on women's health-care issues; she is the author of *The PMS Self-Help Book* (Celestial Arts), *The Menopause Self-Help Book* (Celestial Arts), *Anemia and Heavy Menstrual Flow—A Self-Help Program* (Westchester Publishing), and *Menstrual Cramps—A Self-Help Program* (Westchester Publishing). Individuals who wish to see Dr. Lark for patient care or for lectures and speaking engagements can reach her through *The* LIFECYCLES *Center*. For women who would like more personalized information but live outside the San Francisco Bay Area, she is also available for phone consultation at (415) 964-7268.

Acknowledgment

The author and publisher wish to extend a special acknowledgment to Shelly Reeves-Smith and Cracom Corporation for permission to reproduce the creative line drawings found in the food section of this book. These and additional drawings, together with a collection of wonderful recipes, may be found in the cookbook *Just a Matter of Thyme* available in your local gift or book store. Inquires may be addressed to Among Friends, P.O. Box 1476, Camdenton, MO 65020 or call toll free (800) 377-3566.

Index